PROVIDING FOR THE HEALTH SERVICES

PROVIDING FOR
THE HEALTH SERVICES

Proceedings of Section X (General)
of the
British Association for the Advancement of Science
139th Annual Meeting, 1977

Edited by

SIR DOUGLAS BLACK and G.P. THOMAS

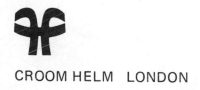

CROOM HELM   LONDON

© 1978 The British Association for the Advancement of Science
Croom Helm Ltd, 2-10 St John's Road, London SW11

British Library Cataloguing in Publication Data

British Association for the Advancement of Science.
  Meeting, Section X (General), 1977
  Providing for the health service.
  1. Medical care – Great Britain – Congresses
  I. Title II. Black, Sir Douglas III. Thomas, G P
  362.1'0941   RA395.G6

  ISBN 0-85664-772-1

Printed and bound in Great Britain

CONTENTS

The 139th Annual Meeting of the British Association for the Advancement of Science was held at the University of Aston in Birmingham from 31 August to 7 September 1977.

The theme chosen by the General Section for discussion at the meeting was 'Investment in Health'; the President of the Section for the Meeting (and the preceding twelve months) was Sir Douglas Black, Professor of Medicine at the University of Manchester and, from 1973 to 1977, Chief Scientist at the Department of Health and Social Security. During his term as President of the Section, Sir Douglas was elected President of the Royal College of Physicians of London.

The Secretary of the General Section of the BA for the 1977 Meeting (and subsequently its Recorder) was Dr G.P. Thomas of the Department of Extra-Mural Studies, University College of Swansea.

1 INTRODUCTION

Sir Douglas Black and G.P. Thomas

The extent of the country's investment in the health and welfare of its population, and how the money set aside for this purpose should be spent, are clearly issues which can never be settled in a way that satisfies everyone. This is especially the case in times, such as the present, of national economic difficulty, and during such times widespread discussion of the questions becomes even more important. It was for this reason, and in the knowledge that a Royal Commission was investigating the future of the National Health Service, that the Committee of the General Section of the British Association chose this area for its discussion in 1977.

The limited time available inevitably meant that only few of the numerous topics suggested could be touched upon, and so, following the general brief of the Section, issues representing widely different parts of the question were given attention. This gave for a varied programme, and hopefully one which reflected the great complexity of health and welfare questions when viewed in a broad perspective.

The papers which follow were presented to the Section at Aston; while small alterations have been made to the original oral contributions, no attempt has been made ruthlessly to eliminate all statements made in the first person singular, indeed it is hoped that their retention will enable readers to appreciate some of the atmosphere of the meeting at Aston.

Following tradition, the first presentation is the Presidential Address by Sir Douglas Black, in which he examines the role of the Department of Health and Social Security in sponsoring research in a number of diverse areas, and outlines some of the difficulties encountered in the post-Rothschild era where the customer-contractor principle operates. These are perhaps particularly apparent in the field of health and personal social services research where liaison between the 'customers' and the 'contractors' drawn from a wide variety of academic disciplines can be established only slowly. Sir Douglas discusses how existing financial constraints accentuate some problems, referring to relations with the Research Councils and to the difficulties of providing tenure in long-term research projects, as particular examples.

Professor Williams' paper refers to the notorious difficulty of

9

defining welfare, let alone of measuring it by conventional economic yardsticks. This inevitably makes judgements of whether a society is generating welfare 'efficiently' very difficult. When these judgements are based on some of the usual classifications of activities as, e.g. productive/non-productive, tradeable/non-tradeable, which are irrelevant in this area, they may even be dangerous. Although there is still a great deal to be achieved, Professor Williams argues that fortunately much broader and more sophisticated views of welfare are now beginning to be reflected in current economic research in this area.

Taking as their targets some of the critics of the NHS and their arguments to the Royal Commission, the Radical Statistics Health Group defend the Service with cogent counter arguments. They suggest, for example, that making people pay directly for their health care would not lead to a more effective use of resources, but could rather distort patterns of medical treatment. They question the powerful position of the medical profession within the NHS and argue that the power of the professionals has an adverse effect on the Service.

The next two papers discuss the roles of two key groups within the NHS, nurses and health visitors, and the arrangements made for their education and training. Professor Altschul looks at recent attempts to define the role of the nurse, attempts which are confounded by the enormous variety of tasks carried out by 'nurses', whether qualified or otherwise. This leads to disagreements as to what would constitute the 'appropriate' education for nursing. Clearly a university-type education which might produce excellent care-organisers at a high level will not be appropriate, or even possible, for the majority of nurses, who undertake the main task of patient care.

Dr O'Connell points to somewhat similar questions in relation to health visitors. The adaptability of the profession over the years has been amply demonstrated by its readiness to assume responsibility for health education and social advice, physical and mental aspects of child development and care, helping the sick and handicapped, and so on. This paper gives a comprehensive account of how the Council for the Education and Training of Health Visitors has set about providing the foundations on which can be built the future success of this many-sided profession.

The National Health Service has been described as a vast oil-tanker – slow to change direction, unresponsive to all but the mightiest pressure. Where does the 'consumer' have a say in how well or wisely the investment is directed on his behalf? Since the reorganisation of the NHS in 1974, the Community Health Councils have a responsibility in this area, and in Pat Gordon's paper their progress and activities so far are charted. Ms Gordon shows how different Councils have interpreted and set about some of the tasks suggested to them, including acting as sources of information both to the public and to the health authorities, and helping individuals with complaints about the NHS.

The next group of papers deals with problems of health raised by the technological basis of our society, and discuss the control of technology in the interests of health. Professor Braun points out the inadequacy of the free market mechanism to exert this control, but suggests that Government-operated incentives or disincentives can be beneficial. Difficult problems remain, particularly in areas of scientific uncertainty; Professor Braun outlines a set of rules which could serve as helpful guides in such situations.

The paper presented by Dr Collingridge and his colleagues compares different strategies that might be adopted for the control of one particular environmental pollutant, lead. Comparisons between strategies are made on grounds of cost-effectiveness, using methods which should be applicable to other pollutants. This method of considering the problem also highlights important gaps in our existing knowledge, which urgently demand increased research effort.

Dr Levy, in his paper, reviews some of the key concepts in the problematic area of occupational cancer and its control, putting the problem in the context of environmentally-induced cancers generally. The difficulties of identifying carcinogenic agents and their threshold limits, if any, are great, and the inadequacies of epidemiological and laboratory investigations are made plain.

About 10 per cent of the annual NHS budget is spent on drugs. The next four papers look at the present use and development of drugs in this country.

Professor Wade asks whether economies in drug use are possible and discusses some ways which have been suggested of encouraging them. These include the provision of incentives or disincentives for the prescriber, regulating the price of drugs, charging the consumer directly, and nationalising the pharmaceutical industry. Professor Wade argues that, whatever the merits or demerits of these various ploys, economy measures of some form are inevitable given the financial constraints on the NHS.

Professor Parish puts drug prescribing in its social context, and examines some of the factors which influence it. He calls for greater communication between the professional groups involved in drug use, puts forward some standards by which responsible prescribing could be judged, and suggests possible solutions for some of the existing problems.

Mr Steward analyses patterns of innovation in the pharmaceutical industry. Recent years have seen rising research costs, stricter safety requirements, more complex scientific problems in the pharmaceutical field, but it is difficult to attribute the decline in levels of innovation to any single one of these factors. Mr Steward argues that 'a substantial proportion of new introductions do not seem to be very useful', while 'uneconomic disease areas tend to be neglected.' Reviewing possible governmental policies, he advocates those which would increase public control over pharmaceutical research and innovation.

Dr Cromie, on the other hand, points to the pharmaceutical industry in the UK as 'a shining example of successful innovation' despite difficulties created by rising costs, over-regulation, anti-vivisection lobbies, and the fact that the UK operates a cheap-drug policy. His spirited defence of the drug companies' oft-criticised information and advertising activities refers to their importance in providing feed-back on responses – adverse or beneficial, to new products. He argues that those who would wish to see the present system changed are putting at risk the population and economy of the UK.

In concluding this brief introduction, we should like to thank all the members of the Committee of Section X of the British Association for their help, and especially Dr Edwin Course of the University of Southampton who, as Recorder of the Section, did so much of the work in making the arrangements for the Aston meeting.

2 RESEARCH FOR WELFARE

Sir Douglas Black

Perhaps the first question that arises in this context is the
deceptively simple one — should research be done? It is sometimes
argued that any available resources should be devoted to the direct
relief of poverty and suffering; and that there is a substantial corpus of
knowledge already in existence, but imperfectly applied. Should more
effort be put into development, even if it would mean a cut-back in
more fundamental research? This is a question which must frequently,
and understandably, arise in the mind of an administrator faced with
the need to make decisions on pressing practical problems. Perhaps
there is some sort of administrative Gresham's law, to the effect that
short-term issues of practicality tend to drive out long-term issues
related to the purposes of a service. My own view, of course, is that this
tempting pragmatic viewpoint is one to be resisted; and a means for
doing so is implicit in the White Paper on Government Research and
Development[1] which recommended that Departments with large
service commitments should include a Chief Scientist's Organisation,
which should both oversee and advocate research into the longer-term
problems of the services provided.

The general case for research may perhaps be illustrated using a
concrete example from the biomedical field. As a house-officer in a
medical ward, I saw many young patients with pneumonia, whose
mortality-rate was 20 per cent, in spite of devoted nursing care; with
the advent, first of sulphonamides, and later of antibiotics, such
patients are now largely treated at home, with a mortality-rate which
is (at least statistically) negligible. There is never, of course, any place
for the sort of complacency which is implied in such phrases as 'the
conquest of infection' -- even in the most successful area, that of
bacterial infections, there are problems of acquired resistance to
antibiotics; and while there are promising leads, viral infections (with
of course the notable exceptions of poliomyelitis and small-pox) remain
relatively 'unconquered'. But the essential point is that discoveries made
in laboratories, whose main function was conceived as the advancement
of knowledge, have from time to time brought about revolutions in
medical care. Of course, elements of chance enter both into the making
of such discoveries, and into their application, so that there is always an

element of risk in research support — one cannot be sure that practical consequences will flow from any particular research proposal. This seems to me the strongest argument which favours a broadly-based and comprehensive approach to research and tells against a narrow mission-oriented tactic. Of course, there comes a later stage, when the basic knowledge has been acquired, at which it may be appropriate to study how it may best be deployed in specific disease states; but the mere existence of a disease state in no way guarantees the success of a frontal attack on a narrow front. Perutz[2] gives examples of the practical application of discoveries, which were apparently made under the stimulus of intellectual interest; and Comroe and Dripps[3] have made a more systematised study of the relative productivity of 'basic' and 'applied' research, which leads them to conclude that 'basic research pays off in terms of key discoveries at least twice as handsomely as other types of research and development combined.'

Medical research has a long history, but it is only within the present century that it can be shown to have had a major impact on the cure of specific disorders. The social and behavioural sciences are of much more recent growth; so it remains to some extent a matter of faith that they will in time make corresponding advances in the cure of social ills. The factors which impair the health of individuals are complex enough; but their complexity is dwarfed by that of the disorders which afflict society. Nevertheless, I am confident that the study of society will in due course (though possibly with a longer lead-time than that of advances in organic medicine) give us more assured techniques for alleviating social malaise. We can learn from the economist, if not how to increase our resources, at any rate how to deploy them more effectively. Psychologists can never teach us too much about human behaviour, and in particular how the appreciation of risks can be made to influence it; again to give a concrete example, teenagers are well informed on the dangers of cigarette-smoking, but this knowledge is little reflected in what they actually do. Management science and social administration have a clear and obvious contribution to make in increasing the efficiency of services; while more fundamental studies in sociology may be able to define objectives, against which we can judge the effectiveness of the services provided.[4] Although the categories may be harder to define, there is clear scope for the development of a social equivalent of the medical epidemiology which is one of the bases of the community approach to health; and the results of this need sophisticated handling by the techniques of statistics and operational research.

These brief remarks hopefully indicate that there is a wide range of research approaches which can bring insights relevant to health and welfare. This now leads to the question of the role of the Department of Health and Social Security in both promoting and benefiting from such research. The Department is responsible for the maintenance of the health and personal social services, and for the provision of social security. These functions are of course to some extent related, and they are also clearly influenced by other social provisions such as housing and unemployment benefit, which are the responsibility of other Departments of Government. Since 1972, the Department has also acquired the responsibility of commissioning biomedical research from the Medical Research Council, to an amount roughly equivalent to a quarter of the Council's total budget, the remainder coming from the Science Vote of the Department of Education and Science.

Types of Research Relevant to DHSS Responsibilities

There are three main areas of research for which the Department now has responsibility — biomedical research; research related to the national health service (NHS) and the personal social services (HPSS research); and research related to the provision of social security.

Biomedical Research

This is the main type of research which is carried out in medical schools, in hospitals and in institutes of medical research; and whose object is to increase our understanding of the factors which maintain human beings in health, as well as those which afflict them in disease. It is a long-established activity of enquiring minds, a part of the general fabric of scientific knowledge. Until the present century, it was carried on either by practising doctors on a part-time basis, or by teachers in the Universities. As Thomson[5] puts it, 'In earlier centuries the advancement of medical knowledge depended on the spontaneous enterprise of men engaged in professional practice and working either in the hospitals or in the general community.' In the early years of this century, it became apparent that further advances were likely to depend to a large extent on the activities of whole-time professional research-workers, who might reasonably look to public funds for their support, since they could not rely on an income from practice. This was a period of remarkable advance in physiology, in some contrast to the virtual inability of physicians to influence the course of disease. It was also becoming appreciated that the provision of funding offered an opportunity for central co-ordination of medical research; and around the same time the National Insurance Act of 1911 set aside a small sum for research. These various strands came together in 1913 with the appointment of the Medical Research Committee, whose first full-time Secretary, the physiologist Sir Walter Fletcher, was appointed in 1916. The new organisation proved its value in the First World War, with important contributions to the treatment of wound shock, to aviation medicine, and to defence against chemical warfare and the epidemics incident to war-time conditions. The Armistice which ended hostilities did not of course do away with medical problems; and in 1920, the Government support for medical research was set on a long-term basis with the establishment of the Medical Research Council. For the next half-century, as described by Sir Landsborough Thomson,[6] the support of medical research from public funds were centred on the Council, which not only set up its own research institutes and establishments, but disseminated medical research throughout the University system by means of training fellowships and various forms of grant support. Medical research is of course supported also in other ways — by the Universities directly; by independent foundations such as the Wellcome Trust and the Nuffield Foundation; and by pharmaceutical and related industry. Nevertheless, the major opportunity and responsibility for a research policy lay with the Council, as indeed it still does. Throughout this long and successful and expanding period of its history, the Council, apart from relatively small private donations and bequests, drew its funds from the Science Vote, a recognition that medical science is part of science as a whole.

There have been some changes in recent years, whose long-term effects are not yet apparent, but which need to be outlined here as they are relevant to the theme of the present address. (Earlier speculations on the effects have been recorded elsewhere.[7]) These changes reflect a belief, widespread among politicians of all parties and also among senior administrators, that Councils composed predominantly of practising scientists (as they must be to have any deep understanding of research) may have a predisposition towards 'scientific excellence' rather than 'social relevance', which is of course a legitimate objective of Government policy. My personal view is that the actual record of activities of the Research Councils gives little support to this belief; nevertheless, it prevailed, and was given formal expression in the White Paper on government research and development.[8] This established a new relationship between the Health Departments and the Medical Research Council, whose main features are the appointment of Departmental nominees on the Council; the transfer of approximately a quarter of the Council's financial support from the Science Vote to the Vote of the Health Departments; and the obligation to administer this Health Department funding in accordance with the customer-contractor principle. It seems to me reasonable in principle that the Health Departments, with their responsibility for the National Health Service and for the Public Health, should have a strong voice in drawing the attention of the Council to priority areas for research. There are, however, great difficulties in deciding on such priorities – should they be based on the burdens imposed by various categories of illness on the NHS; on the needs of client groups; or on the competing claims of pressure-groups, which are often adept at obtaining political support? The changes have certainly led in the short-term to a considerable increase in administrative complexity, which I would hope to see simplified over time. Also, unforeseen shortages of funds, and constraints on the manpower needed to build up the system, have delayed the positive results, the hope of which inspired the White Paper. On the other hand, I am conscious of considerably increased awareness of Departmental need in discussions at the Council and its Boards, as compared with my period on Council as an independent member in the mid-sixties. My own prescription (though like other prescriptions, it may well not be taken) is for an increase in influence, together with a simplification of formal arrangements. Though it is not an easy message to proclaim in times of straitened finance, my experience of the past few years has persuaded me that, as St Paul says, 'the letter killeth, but the spirit giveth life.'

HPSS Research

Whereas the problems of disease and social deprivation go back to the origin of our species, the responsibility of society to meet them in an organised way, in other words the concept of the welfare state, has been clearly recognised only in the present century; and indeed the provision of a national health service and the growth of personal social services, needed to put the concept into practical effect, took place only after the last war.

The heavy cost of these services, and the 'open-ended' character of the problems with which they must deal, have alike raised questions on their efficiency and effectiveness; and wherever there are questions, there are opportunities for research. There are of course, at a high level of generality, qualities which are common to all forms of research – open-mindedness, inventiveness, pertinacity and objectivity. But it would be foolish not to recognise that when it comes to particulars, there are considerable differences between the various fields of research. Not only is HPSS research a new-comer in comparison with biomedical research — it could scarcely have been expected to arise before the services themselves had developed; but it relies on a very different set of scientific disciplines, those related to management and the social sciences. This separation of disciplines is not of course absolute; on the one hand, epidemiology although developed in a medical context, is now making an important contribution in HPSS research, while on the other hand the social and behavioural sciences are becoming increasingly represented in medical training and medical research. The Medical Research Council, while its major interests have remained biomedical, has pioneered research in epidemiology and social medicine; and the increased interest of the Social Science Research Council in health matters is very welcome. Nevertheless, HPSS research looks to a range of University disciplines not found in medical schools — economics, social administration, psychology, social anthropology and sociology. It takes account of the development of University Departments of Nursing Studies; and it derives great benefit from voluntary institutes outside the University system, such as the National Institute of Social Work, the National Childrens' Bureau, the Institute of Community Studies and many others.

Much of the credit for stimulating interest in this important area of research must go to the King Edward's Hospital Fund and the Nuffield Provincial Hospitals Trust, and to comparable voluntary bodies in the field of personal social services. Their initiative has been taken up on a large scale by the DHSS, which is now the major source of funds, and manages a substantial research programme, whose scope and achievements are described in the two volumes of *Portfolio for Health*[9] and in the annual Departmental reports on research and development. There is within the Department a Computer and Research Division, which carries the managerial responsibility for the directly-supported HPSS research programme, as well as for commissioning from the MRC that part of their programme which is funded by DHSS. One of their more difficult tasks is to satisfy the White Paper requirement that 'customer support' must be identified for the research which is being funded by the Department. The 'customers' are representatives of the remaining divisions of the Department — some twenty on the HPSS side alone. These divisions themselves cover large areas of responsibility, whether in terms of 'client groups', such as children, the mentally ill or handicapped, the physically handicapped; or of large services, such as the acute hospital services or primary care. It is far from easy to formulate questions arising from such a wide range of problems, some of which are distinctly 'untidy'; and then to identify research organisations which are competent to tackle them. This very important 'liaison' function of research management between 'customers' and potential 'contractors' is having to be achieved within a framework of accountability, at a time when resources, having expanded rapidly until a few years ago, are now severely constrained. The difficulty of this task is referred to here, not as a curb on the impatience of those who may wish to see everything done at once, but to indicate the importance of fostering relationships of confidence between customers within the Department (for whom research is only one of many preoccupations), and research-workers in the field (who likewise have teaching and administrative responsibilities unconnected with DHSS research).

At this point, the question might well be asked, 'Why has the Department not set up its own "in-house" research facility, recruiting scientists to man it, and thereby evading the need for extensive extra-Departmental liaison work?' Even leaving aside the unacceptability of the increase in civil service manpower which this would entail, there are substantial reasons against it. As has already been indicated, the range of disciplines involved is very wide, and it is clearly more economical to give support to the facilities already established in a number of Universities and other institutes, rather than to attempt to duplicate them. There is the further point that the provision of services is not exactly immune from controversy, in which case there is great merit in the research being carried out by scientists with a standing independent of the Department, even if in a particular context they are funded by it. While support of research extra-murally is the general rule, there are however a few instances in which either a particularly close link with policy, or the need for access to confidential information, makes an in-house facility of a 'mono-disciplinary' type desirable; examples are the Economic Advisers Office and the Operational Research Service of the Department.

Social Security Research

Although the DHSS is responsible for an even greater expenditure on social security than on HPSS, it might seem at first sight that the scope for relevant research is limited, given the combination of statutory rigidity and political sensitivity. This would be a short-sighted view.

Not only are there areas of some flexibility, such as supplementary benefits; but there are also researchable problems related to the take-up of benefits. For example, the legitimate public concern about 'abuse' of benefits has to be seen in this context, that 'those who get money to which they are not entitled are far outnumbered by those who fail to claim benefits to which they *are* entitled'.[10] And in the longer term interests of society, it is surely proper for the DHSS to support research into the causes of poverty, such as we are supporting on commission from the Social Science Research Council.

It is in relation to this sector of the Department's activities that 'in-house' research predominates. The system could not operate at all without the use of computers, and of a very considerable statistical organisation, which constitutes one division of the Department, on the social security side. Within this division, there is a social research branch, whose staff have the necessary access to confidential information. They have explored, or are exploring, the needs of special groups, such as long-stay in-patients in hospital, the bereaved, one-parent families, and those in receipt of invalidity benefit. They are also evaluating an improved claim-form for means-tested benefits. Still within governmental agencies, there is co-operation with the Social Survey Division of the Office of Population Censuses and Surveys (OPCS); with other Departments with related interests; and with the Central Statistical Office, which publishes the very useful annual compilation *Social Trends.* A number of substantial studies are also commissioned from University Departments and other external agencies, on topics such as the long-term unemployed, comparative standards of living, and service for the homeless.

Organisationally, this area of research activity is co-ordinated by a Social Security Research Policy Committee, which includes a number of independent scientists. For the study of specific areas of concern, this body sets up sub-groups; currently, there are two such groups, related to a review of supplementary benefits and to the problems of take-up of benefits.

Departmental Arrangements for Promoting Research

One objective implicit in the White Paper is the involvement in the research programme of a number of advisers with experience in the considerable number of scientific disciplines which have relevance to the categories of research which fall within the Department's responsibilities, whose general character has just been outlined. It is a major responsibility of the Chief Scientist and his organisation to recruit suitable advisers, and bring them into partnership with research management within the Department, and through research management with the policy divisions. A further responsibility of the Chief Scientist is to advise on the balance of the research programme.

This second task is one of some difficulty, in view of the variety of relevant types of research, each of which will have its own advocates; there are the further complications that some parts of the research programme are managed by divisions other than CR division, and that while most of the research is commissioned from the field, some of it is carried on by internal agencies, such as the operational research service and the social research branch referred to earlier. In this part of his task the Chief Scientist is assisted by a Research Committee (the CSRC) whose members are drawn from a number of disciplines ranging from biomedical science to sociology. The members serve for periods up to four years, which allows for some change over time in the disciplines represented, and also gives the members the necessary time to familiarise themselves with Departmental problems. At present, the disciplines represented are biomedical, social medicine, medical administration, administration of personal social services, social administration, nursing studies, psychology and psychiatry, economics and sociology. The executive heads of the Medical and Social Science Research Councils are *ex officio* members, and the total membership is twenty. For the exercise of its 'strategic' role, the committee meets quarterly, one of the sessions being a two-day meeting, the others lasting 4-5 hours.

Important as is the strategic co-ordinating role of advisers on the CSRC, it is also necessary to involve advisers in the research objectives of the various divisions of the Department, which as already mentioned deal with the needs of client groups, or with the provision of particular services. The mechanism devised for this purpose is the Research Liaison Group (RLG), whose components are administrative and professional members of the policy divisions (the 'customers'); members of research management division; and advisers selected for their particular expertise. Some members of the CSRC play a dual role, being also members of RLGs; but it would clearly not be possible to limit the advisers on RLGs to members of the CSRC. The total number of advisers currently serving is 61, but there is considerable variation as sub-groups and working parties are set up to deal with particular areas of concern. There is of course nothing new in the use of advisers — from the inception of the DHSS programme, research applications have been submitted to appropriate referees. What is new is the involvement of advisers in determining the over-all shape of the research programme, as opposed to dealing with particular proposals for research.

In addition to planning its research programme actively to meet perceived service needs, the Department is of course regularly in receipt of proposals for research from workers in the field. The handling of such applications has been formalised by submitting them to a Small Grants Committee, chaired by an independent scientist, and with ten members drawn from a variety of disciplines. As its name implies, this committee deals only with applications up to a ceiling of £30,000, and of a duration not exceeding three years; there is also a 'by-pass', which can be used to channel applications of particular interest to an RLG to that RLG; and the RLGs are also informed of grants awarded in their area of interest.

Before turning to consider some problems in the operation of the system, I must pay tribute both to the willingness of advisers to assist the Department, and to the way in which the various divisions of the Department have been open in considering their advice. At the end of the road, however, the decision rests with the Department, and with the 'customers' therein; but the new arrangements are designed to ensure that the decision should be an informed one, with regard being paid to the scientific feasibility of what is proposed.

Some Problems

One or two of these have already been mentioned – the extent and complexity of the Department's responsibilities, of which in the nature of things research cannot be a major quantitative component; the difficulties which research management, with limited staff, have in securing and formulating a 'customer' view; and the difficulty in deciding on priorities both between and within areas of interest. There are three others which should also be briefly noticed.

The Tenure Problem

The great majority of research-workers employed directly by the Universities and the Research Councils are expected to receive tenured posts after a probationary period of a few years; in contrast to this, research commissioned in strict accord with the customer-contractor principle can only offer a limited prospect of employment. Yet many of the problems relevant to the Department are essentially long-term in nature. In recognition of this, the Department has established a number of units, which are supported on a six-year rolling contract. But while this gives a measure of security to the unit as a whole, it bears hardly on the recruitment of workers, who see alternative prospects of life-long tenure; and it makes it particularly difficult to support the director of a unit (who may himself have a tenured University post) with relatively senior colleagues in 'middle-management'. The present constraints on both the Universities and the Councils make this problem particularly intractable at this time; I regard it as a major disincentive to the development of HPSS research.

Relation with the Councils

Our informal links with the Social Science Research Council raise no particular problem; but the dependence, in part, of the Medical Research Council on the Department for its funding is certainly a potential cause of tension, as was recognised when the transfer of funds was made. This particular decision was taken at a time when the extent and severity of restraints on public spending was not foreseen. The cuts which have since been made have been accepted by the Council, but one must feel sympathy with an organisation which has substantial long-term commitments,but whose funding, coming from two major sources, is insecure.

Constraints on the DHSS

It was originally intended that the RLG system should be progressively extended until all major areas of Departmental research interest were covered in this way. However, the 'spread' of RLGs has been, at least temporarily, cut short for lack of the additional manpower which would be needed to service them; and there are indeed difficulties in servicing even the existing RLGs. Divisions which already have an RLG are at a certain advantage over those which have not; and yet their present distribution, though it reflects to some extent Departmental priorities, can certainly not be firmly equated with them, especially as they may change with changing perceived needs. This has two consequences – it may be necessary to close existing RLGs in order to start others; and the needs of 'non-RLG areas' need particular vigilance. These may of course be temporary difficulties; and in the long-term it may be possible to generalise the RLG system.

Conclusion

In spite of certain difficulties which I have outlined and which are considerably exacerbated by the present restrictions on resources, I believe that the introduction of research advisers on an increased scale, and the involvement of 'customers' in the planning of research, have established a basis on which research funded by the DHSS can be made both scientifically valid and responsive to Departmental needs. There is still a great deal to be done, and important problems to be solved; but we are fortunate in having both an organised system for the delivery of care and welfare, and research-workers who are concerned to study and to improve it. In spite of resource-constraints, the intention of the Department to encourage this important area of research remains firm.

Notes

1. *Framework for Government Research and Development* (Cmd. 5046, HMSO, London, 1972).
2. M.F. Perutz, 'Health and the Medical Research Council', *Nature*, 235 (1972), p.191-2.
3. J.H. Comroe, & R.D. Dripps, 'Scientific basis for the support of biomedical science', *Science*, 192, (1976), p.105-11.
4. The terms 'efficiency' and 'effectiveness' are used here as by Professor A.L. Cochrane in *Effectiveness and Efficiency: random reflections on health services* (Nuffield Provincial Hospitals Trust/Oxford University Press, London, 1972). In this usage, 'effectiveness' relates to the extent to which the objectives of a service are being met; 'efficiency' to those aspects of the *structure* of a service, and of the activities of those employed in it — sometimes summarised as *process* — which decide whether the means employed to achieve these objectives are apt to their purpose, and also economical in manpower and other resources.
5. A.L. Thomson, *Half a century of medical research,* Vol. 1, 'Origins and policy of the Medical Research Council (UK)', Vol. 2, 'The programme of the Medical Research Council (UK)' (HMSO, London, 1973, 1975).
6. Ibid.
7. D. Black, 'Looking at research', *Lancet*, 2 (1976) p.780-4.
8. See note 1.
9. G. McLachlan, *Portfolio for health*, Vols. 1 and 2 (Nuffield Provincial Hospitals Trust/Oxford University Press, London 1971, 1973).
10. D. Donnison, 'Supplementary benefits: dilemmas and priorities', *J. Soc. Policy,* 5 (1976), p.337-58.

3 EFFICIENCY AND WELFARE

Alan Williams

The first difficulty one encounters in talking about efficiency and welfare is that it is not at all clear what 'efficiency' means. And the second difficulty is that it is even less clear what 'welfare' means. These pervasive but elusive concepts underlie a great deal of the business to be transacted by various groups at this 1977 Annual Meeting, particularly where problems of the application of economic notions to social questions are on the Agenda.

This paper discusses some common practical interpretations of what welfare consists of, and the notions of efficiency that go with them. It is argued that however valid some of these notions may be for other purposes, they are of little help if one is trying to determine whether the welfare of the community would be improved if more or fewer resources were allotted to the NHS, or to health care generally or to the public sector at large. This is because commonly used labels such as 'productive' and 'unproductive' cease to have the clear connotations commonly associated with them once one takes a more subtle view of the way in which economic activities contribute to welfare than is contained in the conventions of national income accounting. The order of business is: first to explore the meaning of welfare, then to seek to demolish some simplistic views about efficiency; turning finally to a naive welfare economist's formulation of the problem, and its implications for investment in health.

The Meaning of Welfare

I am now old enough to realise (and even admit) that it is extremely difficult to formulate a comprehensive, unambiguous and operationally meaningful definition of welfare that will be instantly acceptable to all as a working basis for analysis and decision making. But though difficult, it is still important to keep on trying, for although no-one has yet devised the perfect measure, some of the existing ones are more imperfect than others, and we do have some idea of what needs to be done to make them better. What should be done in the fields of health and health service policy will be discussed more specifically later, but initially the problem must be approached at a more general level.

There has been some lively debate over the past decade or so on the extent to which economic growth constitutes, or even contributes to an improvement in general well-being. If, as I believe, economics is about the things that people value, in situations in which they cannot have everything they value, so that they face the necessity of sacrificing some less valuable things in order to gain more valuable things, then I am surprised that there can be any doubt that net growth in the availability of such valuable things is, in the classic phrase, a 'good thing'! The real issue in the economic growth debate is not whether growth is desirable (or possible), but whether it is being measured properly. Put another way, the question that should be asked is 'What is the relationship between welfare and certain key economic variables such as the gross national product, the unemployment rate, the balance of payments, the distribution of income and wealth, and the balance between the public and private sectors?' It is clearly impossible to deal with all these important issues in a paper such as this, but those that are especially relevant to my theme must be tackled.

A National Income Approach

To avoid double-counting, measured national product tries to distinguish items that enter into 'final consumption' from those that are merely used to *produce* items for final consumption. It is not an easy distinction to sustain in practice. For instance that part of private motoring that consists of journeys to and from work is really a cost of production, while that part that consists of sightseeing tours is final consumption. At present many such borderline items are simply treated as 'consumed' including large chunks of investments in consumer durables (other than housing).

In recent years attempts have been made by some economists to identify separately certain items (like defence, police protection, waste disposal and anti-pollution activities) as 'regrettable necessities', which though valuable, are really 'protective', i.e. offsetting the negative side-effects of other activities rather than contributing positively themselves. Although one can sympathise with the motivation of those who seek such refinements, there does not seem to be a very clear cut intrinsic difference between those items which increase social welfare and those which prevent it from declining, for in the last resort one could argue that food is really protection against starvation, housing protection against the elements, entertainments protection from boredom, etc. In any specified circumstance, of course, one can, and should, attempt to evaluate *all* the costs of some recommended measure designed to improve welfare (whether these costs fall on the people promoting the change or not), but the aggregation of these costs, internal and external, into some general welfare index, will surely be beyond us until a large number of these small-scale cost-benefit studies has been done.

As well as items that are counted which some think ought to be reclassified or not counted at all, it is well known that a great deal of valuable economic activity does not even show up in conventionally measured national income — for instance, the services provided by housewives, and a great deal of voluntary activity whether organised through clubs and associations, or whether merely an informed response by individuals or ad hoc groups (e.g. the help of friends or neighbours in domestic or personal crises, large or small).

All this adds up to the casting of considerable doubt as to whether either the level or the direction and extent of change in conventional measures of aggregate economic activity are at all a good guide to what is happening to welfare. It is not surprising, therefore, that attempts have been made to supplement or replace them with various 'social indicators' such as levels of life expectation, morbidity, crime, etc. but so far these have not carried us very far forward, because of the problems of relative valuation which bedevil any system which either cannot, or chooses not to, rely on the market as the source for such valuations. People therefore still tend to fall back on national income statistics, *faute-de-mieux*, and hope that, with all their faults, they will be better than nothing.

The Meaning of Efficiency

When it comes to judging the efficiency of a society in generating improvements in welfare, however, I doubt whether the ideas carried over almost unconsciously from national income accounting really are better than nothing, for their inherent biasses could be seriously misleading. This point may be illustrated by considering the case, recently argued strongly and with widespread publicity for supposing that the way to get Britain out of its present difficulties is to shift resources on a large scale from the public sector to the private sector (and especially to the private *manufacturing* sector). To sustain this case we would need to be convinced that the private (manufacturing) sector will make a greater contribution to the welfare of Britain (at the margin) with the redeployed resources than the sacrifice of welfare entailed when they are taken away from the public sector. (With well over a million employable people unemployed, and an uncertain (but undoubtedly large) amount of our other productive capacity unused, I wonder seriously whether the welfare of Britain might not be more efficiently improved in the short run by concentrating our efforts on measures to eliminate this grossly wasteful margin of unused capacity. My restraint in setting this point on one side is due only to the desire to keep my eyes on our long-term problems, in the none too confident hope that high levels of unemployment are merely a short-term problem.)

Returning to the main argument, my natural instinct would be to look at activities of all sorts, in whatever sector, and range them in order of priority by analysing what good each of them does, for whom, and at whose expense. That is not how the discussion proceeds however. Instead the activities of the society are divided into very broad dichotomous groups, labelled 'productive vs. unproductive', or 'industrial vs. non-industrial', or 'tradeable vs. non-tradeable', or 'marketed vs. non-marketed', and although the distinctions start off by being technical, they end up being perjorative, with the public sector invariably being guilty, by association as it were, with the disliked half of each pair.

Thus productive gets associated with profitable and unproductive with unprofitable, so that activities which do not make profits (e.g. organising transfers from the working to the non-working population) are labelled unproductive and hence seen as a drag on the system, even though all would agree that they improve social welfare. This is due, I am convinced, to the unconscious dominance of the crude GNP model of welfare, which pays no regard whatever to distributional questions.

The industrial vs. non-industrial distinction is even worse, for this harks back to the old idea about primary and secondary sectors, which, at the beginning of the process of industrialisation was used to sustain the view that all material wealth came ultimately from the soil, so that agriculture and mining were the primary sectors, and industry lived parasitically off their output. In the latter stages of the industrialisation process, we now witness the same argument being used by industry vis-a-vis the service sector (private and public), thereby fostering the same backward looking and obscurantist view of economic activity which industrialists themselves had to overcome in Britain two hundred years ago, in which it seems to be denied that on the supply side these different types of activity are complementary and interdependent (i.e. not hierarchical), while on the demand side, their output (tangible or intangible) may be equally valuable to consumers (e.g. I can enjoy a good lecture as much as a trip in a car and as much as a good meal, and the fact that these are in the tertiary, secondary and primary sectors respectively is of no great consequence from a welfare standpoint). I therefore see no basis on these grounds for *presuming* (in the absence of detailed case-by-case analysis) that an intersectoral shift of resources in favour of industry will improve my welfare, or anybody else's.

Let me next consider the distinction between tradeables and non-tradeables, which turns upon whether the goods and services we produce can be sold to foreigners or not. It is clear that services (e.g. shipping, banking, insurance) can be tradeable as well as goods but once one admits the possibility that foreigners can come and live amongst us (as tourists, or students or as temporary residents) it becomes rather difficult to conceive which goods and services are not tradeable. And when we seek to clarify the link between the tradeability of goods and services and their welfare-generating potential, it must rest on the extent to which goods and services that we wish to get from foreigners are worth more to us *at the margin* than the goods and services we are producing ourselves, and this again seems to turn more upon a case-by-case analysis of gains from trade than upon broad distinctions between tradeables and non-tradeables which in any case seem to have little or no meaning.

The final dichotomisation on which I wish to turn a critical eye is that between market and non-market sectors. Useful though this distinction is when one is trying to formulate problems for detailed analysis, I can again see no reason to suppose, prima facie, that it serves as a basis for any general presumptions about the direction in which resources need to be shifted to make the economy more efficient at generating welfare. The market sector includes the entire private sector, and all those nationalised industries that sell their products (which means most of them), provided they do not require subsidies from the state. Here the 'they' is interesting. Is it only nationalised industries that get transmogrified to 'non-market' status if they run deficits, or is the agricultural sector non-market too on account of our agricultural subsidy system? Can the substantial tax allowances for investment enjoyed by manufacturing industry, etc. be distinguished analytically from state subsidies, and, if not, exactly who is left in the market sector? At this point there seem two possible ways forward. Either one says 'to the extent that the sector is non-market this will happen' in which case we need detailed analysis of the situation, *or* the argument degenerates into an entirely different set of propositions about tax burdens on the 'productive' (or profitable) in order to support the 'unproductive' (or unprofitable), and in this way we come full circle and are back where we started.

A Welfare Economics Approach

I hope that by now I have convinced you of the obscurity, sterility and irrelevance of these arguments if one's interests are in judging how to increase welfare (rather than how to increase conventionally measured GNP). I would prefer to divide economic activities into those which contribute to welfare immediately (labelled consumption) and those which should contribute to it in the future (labelled investment) and to recognise that most activities, in all sectors, have the potential to be in either category.

I would call an activity unproductive only if it contributed to neither, and there are doubtless examples of unproductive activities in all sectors, and the proper pursuit of efficiency requires them to be stopped and the resources redeployed more productively. I cannot see that labelling an activity unprofitable necessarily condemns it from a welfare viewpoint, although it will be condemnatory in the eyes of those who were induced to part with money in the expectation that it would earn them returns over and above their cash investment. Nor can I see any great welfare gain by making goods more tradeable, since tradeability seems to me a morally neutral attribute.

Greater marketability, on the other hand, I could conceive of as being morally reprehensible, if it implied (as it surely would) that some goods and services (e.g. access to health care) which are at present largely allocated by non-market criteria were to be redistributed in favour of those with greater market power. It is disappointing that the enormous increase in sophistication in the analysis of markets which has been the major contribution of welfare economists in the past 20 years has still made so small an impact on those who persist in arguing in terms of grand national accounting aggregates.

Implications for Health and Health Care

In the limited conception of welfare that relates essentially to GNP, health is important for the 'productive' members of the society, but something of a luxury for the rest, and access to health care should be allocated accordingly if it is itself to be productive. No reputable economist working in the health field would subscribe to that view, though it would be equally foolish and erroneous to deny that if health care does improve productivity in this narrow sense, that is, as far as it goes, a 'good thing'. But it is not the only 'good thing' that can come from health care. Good health is enjoyable for its own sake. It improves the quality of life generally, whether for working or for leisure activities. Although the goods and services required for the enjoyment of certain kinds of leisure enter into GNP, leisure time itself does not, yet it is a considerable contributor to welfare, and one which good health can greatly extend. In this broader sense, health care directed to the elderly can be as productive (of welfare, if not of GNP) as health care directed to the working population. It is a matter of maintaining the appropriate balance at the margin, and not a matter of extolling the one *in toto* and condemning the other in equally aggregate terms.

I do not want to suggest, however, that good health depends largely on access to health care. Health is like a stock of capital with which we are initially endowed, and which naturally depreciates through time, and at an increasing rate in later life. Within limits we can diminish or augment this personal capital stock by our general lifestyle. Eating, drinking, smoking and worrying too much will run down our capital, just as will too little exercise, and we may then turn to the health service to make good these depredations, which it certainly has some (severely limited) capacity to do. So health care can be seen as improving our immediate well-being (i.e. our current consumption) and as improving our future well-being by arresting the rate of depreciation of our stock of health capital, and in this sense it is a consumer durable. If we are wise, we will not rely on it to do the whole job for us, however.

Current economic research into health care does fortunately reflect this much broader view of 'welfare' when judging the 'efficiency' of health services, and this broadening has had the further beneficial effect of enabling economists to link their work more effectively with that of epidemiologists and other medical researchers who have been (and to some extent still are) suspicious of our supposedly blinkered approach. This is not to imply that all is now sweetness and light in this difficult territory. One still does not gain instant popularity by insisting that the fact that some medical treatment will do someone somewhere some good is not enough to justify providing facilities immediately to do it. Before the latter conclusion can be accepted, one has to be convinced that no other use of those same resources will do anyone anywhere *more* good. Indeed, the golden rule is that only when we can be satisfied that the *most* valuable thing that we are *not* doing, is less valuable than the *least* valuable thing that we *are* doing, can we be sure that we are being efficient in the pursuit of welfare. I guess we have a long way to go yet.

4 IN DEFENCE OF THE NATIONAL HEALTH SERVICE

Radical Statistics Health Group

Introduction

It is apparent that the basis of the National Health Service (NHS) is under attack from a number of influential groups in this country[1]. Many of these groups have taken the opportunity presented by the Royal Commission on the NHS to put forward proposals that would fundamentally damage the service. In our 'defence of the NHS'[2] we have examined in detail some of the proposals made to the Royal Commission about the financing of the NHS and show how their implementation would positively harm the service and challenge the basis on which it was founded.

Two kinds of argument are commonly used to justify changes in the financing of the health service. The first is that the provision of health care which is free at the time of need encourages excessive use of the service. The second argument, which follows from the first, is that it is impossible to provide adequate financing for the health service entirely from public funds.

Evidence about these suppositions is often based on anecdotal accounts of experiences in this country and elsewhere and on a comparison of total health care expenditure in different countries with differing methods of health care organisation. We have summarised the position in some of these countries, and on this basis we have refuted both arguments. Making people pay for their health care does not necessarily discriminate between 'real' and 'unreal' need, nor help them to make more effective use of the health service. In fact, the methods of insurance which inevitably accompany 'fee for service' medicine lead both to higher administrative costs and a distorted market for items of medical care.

Simply comparing our expenditure on health with the greater expenditure in other countries does not prove that we spend too little. In fact, such comparisons frequently indicate that the overall health of a population is more closely related to their standard of living than to the percentage of the Gross National Product allocated to health. To establish that the NHS is inadequately financed requires convincing evidence that spending more money will result in some measurable

33

improvement in the physical and mental health of the people, and that this improvement is greater than that which could be achieved by alternative ways of spending the money.

Paying for Medical Care

In the first place the various methods which have been proposed to increase the revenue of the NHS may be considered. These include fee for service payments for items of medical care given, such as fees for visits to General Practitioners, cost-related prescription charges and hospital hotel charges. The private health insurance schemes which are proposed to pay for these changes also must be considered here. By taking examples from various other countries where such payment schemes are in operation, it can be demonstrated that they inevitably distort medical practice and accentuate inequalities in health care.[3] In addition, we have examined the British dental service, where fee for service payments are used and shown that this piecework system encourages over-hasty work and concentration on the more profitable treatments to the detriment of adequate preventive dentistry.[4]

Private Medicine and Other Attacks on the NHS

In order to understand the context of the proposals on alternative financing for the NHS we have examined the motives behind them. We suggest that these proposals have been put forward by people who are keen to provide a service mainly for certain elite sections of society, and to support the development of private practice for vicarious reasons.

The damaging effects of the continuation of private practice within the NHS are documented. We discuss the parasitic nature of the private sector on the NHS[5] and the way in which it threatens the continuation of the health service in its present form. We argue that any significant expansion of the private sector will seriously threaten the basis on which the NHS was created and therefore lead to a worse provision of health care to most people. The concept of freedom of choice is briefly discussed and its real meaning examined in the context of health care. The issue of freedom of choice, put forward as a positive benefit of private medical systems, is an attempt to give the private sector an appearance of concern with human rights. At the same time, this diverts attention from the low level of general knowledge about health, and the need for more democratic control over the health service as presently organised. Those who seem so concerned about freedom of choice when trying to justify the making

of profits from medical care are rarely heard to demand greater
freedom of choice within the NHS.

What about the Effectiveness of Medical Practice?

It is known that there are many areas within the NHS where health
care could be improved without additional financing, and other
areas where money could be saved without detriment to the patient.
As this knowledge has obvious relevance to and implications for any
discussion of alternative financing we continue with an examination
of the effectiveness of some aspects of medical practice. In particular,
we concentrate on some common surgical procedures because they
constitute a part of medicine where the opportunities for private
practice are greatest and where the amount of intervention varies most
according to the method of medical care organisation.

We concentrate on five operations which account for about
one-quarter of all surgical procedures. In the NHS the frequency of
these operations does not vary very much between different areas of
Britain but they are generally more common in the United States
and Canada.[6] In some instances, they are four or five times more
common in these countries and the variation between different areas
in North America is usually greater than the variation between areas
in the UK. Differences in neither disease patterns nor age
composition between these countries are sufficient to explain such
marked differences in these rates of surgery. For example, the
probability of an American citizen undergoing any surgery is nearly
twice as high as that for an English citizen. It is not possible to argue
from that fact which rate is the more appropriate in terms of the effect
it has in improving the health of the community, because it is not
known what would be the consequences of doubling the surgery
rate here or halving the rate in America. Outcome measures with
which this question could be answered are only usually obtained
without bias from controlled trials where people are randomly
allocated to surgery or some alternative treatment (e.g. no treatment).

However, close examination of the difference in these rates appear
to be associated with a high density of surgeons and in particular with
the method of payment for surgery. Where people contract with a
Health Maintenance Organisation (HMO) for a fixed annual fee to
look after all their medical care needs, the rates are more
comparable with those of England and Wales. Where people pay via
some insurance cover on a fee for service basis the rates are closer to
the prevailing national US rate. Therefore one can conclude that the

discretion of both the referring doctor and the surgeon must be large and that non-medical considerations play an inappropriate part in the decision of whether or not to operate.

For some procedures the amount of discretion is naturally limited by pathological evidence. For instance, a breast is rarely surgically removed unless examination of a sample of tissue indicates strongly that cancer is present. Therefore one might expect that the variation in the rate of Mastectomy was relatively less than some procedures for which little useful pathological evidence existed. It is shown in Figure 1 of the pamphlet that the rates for fee for service medicine are four times higher than for HMO's for tonsillectomy, twice as high for Hysterectomy and Inguinal hernia repair but only one and a half times as high for Mastectomy. Moreover, the prevalence of the more radical (and therefore more expensive) treatment for breast cancer is four times higher in the US and Canada than in the UK whereas all clinical trials comparing radical mastectomy with simple mastectomy fail to demonstrate a difference in therapeutic usefulness.[7]

Evidence about the effectiveness of the other surgical procedures is discussed and it is shown that many commonly performed operations seem to make little measurable difference (one way or the other) to the well-being of those subjected to them.[8] They do, however, cost money. But this criticism also applies to many of the other areas of medical care which we characterised by surgical, technological or pharmaceutical interventions. Contrary to the popular image of a scientifically-based medical profession, the reality is that relatively few of the techniques used by doctors have been evaluated in a scientific manner before becoming generally used. Occasionally, the dangers or benefits of an innovation are so obvious that they are promptly and unanimously recognised. More often, conflicting views exist with the result that individual doctors use treatments to a varying extent[9] and in varying circumstances. Thus the doctor's concept of his inalienable right to 'clinical freedom' is used to justify the entirely unethical situation in which he subjects his patients to uncontrolled experimentation with techniques which have not been scientifically evaluated.

The Medical Profession

We conclude with a discussion of the medical profession. Doctors continue to be the most powerful group within the health service and we discuss the obvious manifestations of their hegemony and how it is maintained. In particular, we discuss the concept of clinical freedom, its role in the provision of health care and role of the profession in its protection by examining the prescription of drugs in the NHS.[10]

The moulding of the aspirations of medical students to the ideology of the profession is an important part of the power of the profession. As would be expected, after a large number of years in the inappropriate atmosphere of one of the large teaching hospitals, many young doctors emerge with identical values and similar career preferences to those who selected and trained them. After qualification the doctors are keen to protect their status and practise technological medicine without any form of control rather than working to meet the real needs.

Conclusions

Finally, we are of the opinion that the NHS and the patterns of health care delivery can only be a mirror and example of the patterns of distribution of other resources within our inequitable society. However, we believe that the NHS offers a method of medical care organisation which provides as equitable and just a provision for medical needs as is possible within these constraints of our society. The purpose of the foundation of the NHS in 1948 was to 'promote the establishment of a comprehensive health service, redesigned to secure improvements in the physical and mental health of the people and the prevention, diagnosis and treatment of illness'. It is free (apart from some exceptions) and available to everyone in the country. These are fundamental principles on which to base the organisation of medical care.

We do not assert that the NHS is faultless or incapable of improvement. However, we do argue that before proposals for change which ignore these basic principles can be allowed serious consideration, a heavy burden of proof of their effectiveness, in terms of the original purpose of the NHS, will be necessary.

Notes

1. BMA, 'Evidence to the Royal Commission on the National Health Service', *BMJ*, 1, p.314.
2. Radical Statistics Health Group, *In Defence of the NHS* (RSHG, c/o 9 Poland Street, London, W1V 3DG, 1977).
3. Brook, R.H. and Avery, A.D., 'The US Scene' in *A Question of Quality* (Nuffield Provincial Hospital Trust, OUP, 1976).
4. Dental Estimates Board — *Annual Reports 1970-75* (Eastbourne).
5. Norfolk Area Health Authority, *Financial Returns* (1976).
6. E. Vodya, 'A Comparison of Surgical Rates in Canada and England and Wales,'

38 In Defence of the National Health Service

New Eng. J. Med., 289 (1973), p.1224.
7. J.P. Binker, 'Surgical Manpower', *New Eng. J. Med.*, 282, (1970), pp.135-44.
8. K. McPherson and S.F. Fox, 'Treatment of Breast Cancer' in J.P. Binker, B.A. Bones and F. Mosteller (eds), *Costs, Risks and Benefits of Surgery* (OUP, 1977).
9. J.P. Binker, B.A. Bones. and F. Mosteller (eds.), *Costs, Risks and Benefits of Surgery* (OUP, 1977).
10. A.L. Cochrane, *Effectiveness and Efficiency* (Nuffield Provincial Hospitals Trust, 1972).
11. *Report of the Committee of Enquiry into the Relationship of the Pharmaceutical Industry with the NHS* (1965), (Cmnd. 3410 HMSO, 1967).

5 EDUCATION AND ROLE OF NURSES

A.T. Altschul

In 1972 a report[1] was published by the 'Committee on Nursing', a committee set up in 1970 under the Chairmanship of Professor Asa Briggs, 'to review the *role* of the nurse and the midwife in the hospital and the community and the *education and training* required for that role, so that the best use is made of available manpower to meet present needs and the needs of an integrated health service'. The title of this paper is thus allied to the remit of the 'Briggs' Committee, but does not of course constitute a résumé of the findings of the Briggs Committee nor does it propound a comprehensive alternative solution to the vexed problem of role and education of the nurse.

It may seem strange to non-nurses that we should be preoccupied, year after year, to define our role when, it would appear, other professionals do not find it necessary to do so. The Briggs Committee, referring to opinions expressed to them, said they agreed that:

1. the role of the nurse must always be closely related to the needs of the patients;
2. these needs are never static but vary according to individual patients, medical and technical advances and developments, such as the possibility of a unified nursing service; and
3. that this changing role can never be considered adequately in isolation from the role of other members of the National Health Service.

The Committee's brief was confined to the examination of nursing in relation to the National Health Service. If we wish to go beyond it, for example within the United Kingdom to the role of those nurses who do not work within the National Health Service, or if we try to understand the role of the nurse in other countries, we must add a fourth point to the list, namely that:

4. the nurse's role depends on the nature of the health care system within which patients are cared for.

39

This role will be different in private practice from that in the hospital ward, different in countries where most patients pay, from the role in a country where few do so.

If any headway is to be made in understanding the role of the nurse, a definition of those workers to whom we wish to apply the label 'nurse' must first be attempted. By law the title 'nurse' is restricted (a) to those whose names are on a register or roll of one of the General Nursing Councils and (b) to those on an index of student nurses or a list of pupil nurses.

It would be easy to count nurses on the registers or rolls of the Councils if England and Wales had not decided to make registration a permanent status, resulting in far more names on the register and roll than are actually practising; whereas in Scotland a live register is maintained by requiring nurses to renew their registration annually. It is, however, possible to work in Scotland while registered in England, so that in Scotland the size of the current register underestimates the numbers of practising nurses. Either way the number of learners in nursing at any one time is much larger than the number of qualified practising nurses. Yet to discuss their role separately is meaningless as their main function should be to prepare themselves for their future role as qualified nurses.

Patients and other members of the public who are potential patients tend to think of student nurses when they are asked to define the nurse's role as it appears to them or, more commonly still, they think of auxiliaries who are not nurses at all but only helpers to nurses. They may do valuable work and be highly respected people, but they are not nurses, though their numbers count on the pay-roll of the nursing staff. We are providing for patients a system of nursing care which is predominantly carried out by people who are not qualified nurses, namely by students, pupils and auxiliaries.

Some important questions can now be raised. For instance, should we accept the situation in which nursing care is delivered by non-nurses and concentrate on the organisational role of the qualified nurse who has to be responsible for the work of non-nurses? Would the quality of care be better if it were carried out by nurses? Could it ever come about that care would be administered by qualified nurses only? Would it be more expensive than it is now, and, most importantly in relation to the topic under discussion, would a different scheme of education be required if nurses were educated to nurse and not, as now, to organise, supervise and control the care given by non-nurses.

Let us indulge in a little simple arithmetic to calculate what the staffing requirements may be in the case of hospital care, bearing in mind that nurses also work in the community and in many other situations in which their professional training may not be immediately recognised as relevant, for example as journalists, as researchers, as factory or school nurses.

Supposing in a hospital ward four nurses were needed at any one period during the day and night. The week has 672 hours. Nurses work 40 hours per week at the moment; they are trying to reduce this to 35 hours per week. The hospital would have to employ 16¾ nurses at 40 hours per week each to provide 4 on each shift in one week, not allowing for any overlap or for fluctuations which may result from the constraints imposed by meal breaks or other off-the-ward activities. Because overlaps are important for effective communication and because of holidays and sickness, several more are in fact required for such a ward. Would it really make sense to define the role of each of the 16¾ nurses? Would it not make more sense either to define only the role of *one* nurse, namely the role of the one who takes charge of all 16¾ nurses, or to abandon the quest for role definition altogether and to make explicit instead the total care requirements of each patient, leaving one or more people to attend to the distribution and supervision of the work of nurses or non-nurses, according to their competence and personality?

In the first case we have to decide what education is necessary to enable the nurse to perform her organisational, administrative function in relation to team work of a complex clinical nature. In the second case we must attempt to establish whose professional role includes the organisation and supervision of the work of others, be they professional or non-professional. In this country, ever since Florence Nightingale, it has been customary for nurses to be responsible for the organisation and delivery of care which, at the time, is regarded as nursing care. In the past such care included the necessary domestic work, the provision of food, the ordering of hardware stores and of equipment. In the care of mentally ill patients it included the supervision of patients' work and leisure and the training of patients for work or for social living. Currently a large proportion of these responsibilities have been taken over by others, for example by domestic staff, occupational therapists, teachers or social workers. In some countries all of the organisation is seen to be part of the role of the doctor, who feels personally responsible for the training of every helper whom he calls nurse.

It seems clear then that much of the disagreement which exists about the role and education of the nurse hinges on the fact that it has never been defined to which worker the label 'nurse' should be applied. If it is to be applied to each of the 16¾ nurses in my example, then the role is a low level one for which almost anyone can be recruited and trained. The Briggs Committee in fact states that in nursing there is room for everyone with from low average to high ability.

If the title nurse is to be given to all staff who fall under the command of the doctor, the role must be a low level one, as no-one capable of higher level functioning is likely to accept permanent subservience to doctors.

It the label 'nurse' is to be applied to the persons who are responsible for the total nursing work of say 16¾ people, the education of the nurse must reach a high level of conceptual thinking, enabling the nurse to fulfil a forward planning, policy making role in relation, not only to 16¾ nursing personnel, but also in relation to interdisciplinary communication, team work and care planning. At the highest level in the National Health Service at the moment the chief nurse shares as an equal the responsibility for the delivery of care with the doctor and the administrator. She/he is responsible for the work of several thousand members of the nursing staff and for a budget of, in one area, £37½ million. The high level function of such a nurse can only be carried out if, in the first instance, candidates of high ability are recruited to nursing and if at every stage of her career, work of high level competence and responsibility is expected of the nurse.

The Briggs Committee suggest that the role of the nurse depends on the patient's needs. I should like to add that it depends on the patient's perception of his needs and on his interpretation of the nurse's role. If, for example, the patient has a need for a bedpan, but he regards the role of trained nurses as being above providing a bedpan, he will not express his need to the nurse and consequently reinforce the attitude that the bedpan-giving is not part of the role of the nurse. If the patient needs a willing listener, whether or not he perceives this to be the role of the nurse will contribute to the role definition the nurse creates for herself.

On the whole patients resolve the conflict they experience in role definition of nurses by regarding nursing as the function of the nursing staff collectively without specifying which aspect of nursing care they allocate to each member of the nursing staff. This diffuse role definition at times suits nurses very well as it permits them to work in a system of job allocation which can incorporate trained and untrained personnel, which divides responsibility and thereby reduces accountability, which allows nurses to claim the prestige due to them because they are collectively always present and concerned with every aspect of patient care, but at the same time legitimates the delivery of only minimal care because the high ideals of total patient care for everyone cannot be realised.

I have now shown that indeed, as Briggs says, the nurse's role depends on four factors:

1. patient's expressed needs and his identification of these needs as 'nursing needs';
2. on technological and scientific advance in so far as this can be comprehended by the nurse;
3. on the aspects of care which other professions claim as their role, for example, occupation, speech, mobility or social problems;
4. on the decision whether each nurse is a professionally responsible person or whether the collective activities of all nurses are the responsibility of a member of their own or some other profession.

Before we move on to consider in more detail the education of nurses, I should like, briefly, to remind readers that in the United Kingdom the General Nursing Councils maintain not one, but four Registers of Nurses, one for general nurses, the others for sick children's nurses, mental nurses and, in England and Wales, nurses for the mentally subnormal, in Scotland for the mentally defective. While most people feel that they intuitively understand the role of the general nurse, there are many who do not find it easy to conceptualise the role of the nurse in relation to the mentally disordered. If they describe such nurses as 'not real nurses' they take their own image of the general nurse as one about whose role consensus exists; but we have already shown that this is far from the truth. Add to the questions we have already asked such questions as — what are the common elements of care or of the underlying science which lead us to use the label 'nurse' for workers with such dissimilar roles? What room is there in the care for the mentally disordered for qualified nurses and unqualified helpers? What other professional people are needed in the care of the mentally disordered person? — and you will appreciate how difficult it is to find an educational process which might be deemed appropriate to the development of 'the nurse'.

I have described a series of dichotomies in the roles of nurses. If the premise is accepted that we either call the person who delivers basic care 'the nurse' or the person who organises basic care, it follows that

for the former role there is a need for on-the-job training, perhaps
with subsequent in-service education aiming at incremental
competence. It also follows that for the latter role selection must take
place from candidates with high ability and intelligence, that for such
learners an education must be provided which is interesting,
challenging and demanding. Whether or not nursing needs university
graduates might be debatable; what is certain is that it needs people
who are capable of profiting from university education and in the
current educational climate we can only recruit such people if we
provide university education for them.

We can now try to find out whether we have any choice in
assigning high or low level roles to the people labelled 'nurse' and
whether we are free to plan an educational programme accordingly.
I would suggest that we have very little scope in this respect. To
become a nurse is the aim of very many young people and in their
plans the educational hurdles do not present either incentives or
obstacles. Teachers and parents alike regard nursing as a career for the
less able pupils. They must be gradually persuaded that nursing also has
a great deal to offer for the brightest pupils. While we slowly penetrate
into universities, we must maintain the starry-eyed interest of the
majority who will enter nursing at a less demanding level. Again I
should like to quote the Briggs report: 'At the point of entry to the
nursing and midwifery profession, applicants should be drawn from a
wide range of intelligence from average to the highest. Suitability
should not be determined by O levels alone'.

The suggested 'modular' system of training, leading via a low level
certificate of nursing to registration and to higher certificates, is
designed to bring all learners into the profession through a common
portal of entry but to permit all who wish to do so to add to their
knowledge and experience in order to raise to a higher level their
role and function. We could not, in this country, elect to hand over
responsibility for nursing education to the medical profession,
because their knowledge of nursing has been allowed to wither while
nursing undertook the training of its own professionals. We must,
therefore, educate at least some learners for their subsequent role
as teachers and managers at ward sister level, nursing officer level or
above.

We could not educate all nurses, however, in colleges of higher
education, such as technical colleges or universities. If we tried to do so,
bearing in mind the many thousands of learners entering nursing each
year, universities or colleges of technology would have no space or

resources left for the teaching of any other subject.

The National Health Service is geared to the employment, cheaply, of learners who shoulder the main workload of patient care. The financial implications for the Health Service, if all nurses were to be educated in educational institutions outside the Health Service, would be colossal. But of all health professions nursing alone has allowed itself to be deprived of properly organised education. Even the future helpers to physiotherapists, occupational therapists and staff of homes providing residential care are now being trained under the educational umbrella. In some countries, Sweden and Australia for example, effort is now being made to take nursing education out of the Health Service. We would need at least some nurses in universities, even if the majority were educated in the colleges of education and technology, because progress in nursing and improvement in care will ultimately depend on teaching nurses to do research and on putting research findings into practice. Universities are still, in this country, the right milieu for research.

We have no choice then, in this country, but to continue educating nurses in hospital-based schools of nursing, in technical colleges and in universities, but we should remember that the output is of very different practitioners with only the title 'nurse' in common.

We must remember, however, that the British holders of the title 'nurse' may want to compare themselves with their counterparts elsewhere. In some countries, notably on the continent of Europe, they will find doctors firmly in charge of nurse training and the practising nurses well below themselves in status. In the USA and Canada they will find their counterparts, to a much larger extent, university educated. In some parts of the USA nearly 50 per cent of all school leavers proceed to universities. Future nurses obviously must be included in that top half of the population.

In some developing countries too they will find nurses with university education. Where only a small percentage of people is literate, a high proportion of these proceed to university. Nurses need to be able to read and it is, therefore, appropriate for them to join in the student body of the land. There, however, the title 'nurse' is reserved for those who are responsible for teaching and managing others. Those who give direct care do not aspire to the title. They are health care workers locally recruited and trained and locally respected and trusted. The system of patient care in which not everyone who gives nursing care is a nurse is worthy of further study.

Changes in the role and education of nurses are inevitable. It may be apposite to examine the many contradictory roles which nurses now display and to make rational decisions about the future of the profession and the education of its practitioners rather than to continue to allow random development and diversification to take place.

Note

1. *Report of the Committee on Nursing* (Cmnd. 5115, HMSO, London, 1972).

6 THE PROFESSIONAL EDUCATION OF HEALTH VISITORS AND THEIR ROLE IN HEALTH CARE

Patricia E. O'Connell

There are few professional roles which have proved more difficult to define and describe than that of health visiting. This is partly because of its broad range of activity, partly because by nature the public health nurse of the past has been self-effacing and inarticulate about her own work, and partly because the results of the health visitor's work are difficult to measure. A 'nutshell' definition of the service is that health visiting is the preventive arm of the community nursing service. The difficulty in evaluating success arises from the negative measurement involved. Success in preventive health activity is measured by absence of disease and disorder. It is only over a long span of time, and with the use of vital statistics collected over decades, that improvement in health and absence of disease becomes evident. And even then how far is it possible to select aspects of improvement in health patterns and attribute them to the work of one profession, when advances in housing, social conditions and the scientific aspects of health studies run parallel?

Health visiting has never stood alone in its development. As a profession health visitors have been influenced by contemporary trends which related to employment of women and patterns of general and professional education. The character of their work has been influenced by the needs of the society they were called upon to serve and the social and scientific tools which were available at the time. Health visitors are nothing if not adaptable. Frequently their work has accrued according to changing requirements of a public medical/social service, and often work initiated by health visitors as part of a general function has later become the prime focus of a new profession. A notable example of this is the child care service which, in pre-Curtis-Committee days, was staffed on the child life protection side by health visitors. This later passed to specialised child care officers in a co-ordinated service of day and residential care for children deprived of normal home life.

A brief survey of approximately a century of public health care (now more commonly called community health care) will suffice to trace the field of work of health visitors. Once this has been outlined their role and function become easier to discuss.

In the late nineteenth century public health was concerned with sanitary health and hygiene and the early health visitors, traditionally associated with the Manchester and Salford Ladies Sanitary Reform Society in 1862, worked among deprived and ill-educated families plying them with tracts on cleanliness if they could read and packets of disinfecting powder if they could not. Organised by the lady charitable workers of the period, the actual visitors were described as 'respectable working women' whom it was felt would relate easily with the clients they served. With the birth of epidemiology as a science and the rise of the philanthropic child welfare movement in the late nineteenth century, the medical aspects of health and sanitary care started to predominate and a worker with more scientific and practical knowledge was sought.

This was the period when Florence Nightingale was concerning herself with the standards of the nursing profession, when Elizabeth Blackwell achieved her medical degree as the first woman to qualify, and when the midwifery profession was being organised under the Central Midwives Board in 1902. In fact the professional woman was emerging as a trained, responsible worker ready to be harnessed for the public service. The need for training was recognised although social service was still largely organised under the auspices of voluntary action. At this stage health visiting work was associated almost exclusively with maternity and child welfare and the most appropriate basic qualification lay in medicine, midwifery or nursing. After some experimentation, in which the Huddersfield Birth Notification scheme featured importantly, the most appropriate qualification for the health visitors was found to be basically nursing and midwifery to which specialised public health nursing training was attached.

In the early twentieth century when the school health service developed, school nursing found a parallel to health visiting and in many cases one woman carried out both functions in a vicinity. With the development of the dispensary system for the treatment of Tuberculosis, the preventive work in this service was also based on health visiting so that during the inter-war years, 1918 to 1939, there emerged a worker, employed by local health authorities or voluntary associations who carried out preventive work for the mother and young child as a health visitor, for the school child as school nurse, and for the full age range in Tuberculosis care and prevention. Local authorities employed a given number of such workers on the staff of the Medical Officer of Health and each was responsible for a geographical area of the authority, working from health department or clinic premises. In the more rural parts of the county where the population was more scattered and services less sophisticated the role of health visitor, district nurse and midwife was vested in one worker who operated from her own house and over the whole range of preventive and curative nursing. Such a combined or 'triple-purpose' nursing service was frowned upon by many because the conflicting priorities of child-birth, sick nursing and health education often led to neglect of the preventive role.

In 1948 with the introduction of the National Health Service, the range of health visiting functions was broadened to include care of the whole family from the 'cradle to the grave'. Added to her responsibility for mother and children was that of 'care and aftercare in the case of illness'[1] and health education of the whole family. Because of the change in population structure and the increased awareness of the needs of the elderly, health visitors found that there accrued to them a caseload of elderly, frail and lonely who needed preventive work and health care in their own homes. Because of the advance in medical science and the consequent survival of many handicapped who previously died at birth or soon after, the health visitor was called upon to counsel and support many parents and relatives who were caring for handicapped children and adults.

This breadth of caseload increased the interest of the work and brought into play the health visitor's nursing skills to a greater extent than previously. However it raised a number of difficulties. Firstly the very breadth of work created confusion in those who made calls upon the service. The WHO definition of health alluded to its 'physical, mental and social aspects' and in this context there is only a fine divide between the functions of health visiting and social work. Both health visitors, their employers and their clients needed some guidance as to role and function and only when both aspects had been defined was it possible to consider appropriate specialist education and training.

In 1953 the Jameson working party was set up by the Ministry of Health and the report 'An Inquiry into Health Visiting' was published in 1956.[2] In this report the function of health visitors was defined as 'health education and social advice' and her field of work was confirmed as extending over the full age range of the population but only in the preventive sphere. Other studies should be 'incidental' to this, her prime function. Combined district nursing and health visiting was to be discouraged, but at the same time a new association between health visitor and general medical practitioner was seen to be desirable. In its recommendations the working party quoted the GP as 'tending to become the clinical leader of the domiciliary health services team'. It saw the health visitor as being 'admirably placed to help him. She could be useful to him in any part of his practice where health education and social advice are desirable' (Para. 305-7). In summary, 'in the ordinary course of her work and without exceeding her competence, she could be in a real sense a general purpose family visitor' (Para. 314-16).

The health visitor's advisory role in the maternity and child welfare field had been predominately concerned with physical health and Jameson emphasised the need to give equal weight to mental aspects of development and care. This was in keeping with the health philosophy of the era when the importance of mental and emotional health was for the first time being given the attention it merited.

Having defined the work of health visitors the Jameson Committee made recommendations about training. It confirmed the view that the basic professional requirement for health visiting was general nursing and some obstetric preparation. A central training council was envisaged and some general guidance on syllabus and examination was offered. By 1962 a similar, if more weighty, report on social work and its training needs had emanated from the Younghusband Committee[3] and as a result the Health Visiting and Social Work (Training) Act was passed. This set up two training councils for the two professions and linked them by means of a common chairman and some common membership. However, separate training arrangements were made and these brought unequal expansion of the two professional training bodies. As a result it was expedient to separate the two councils on implementation of the LAS Services Act in 1972. At this stage the health visitor council assumed a new title 'The Council for the Education and Training of Health Visitors' (CETHV) and a separate chairman was appointed for eacn of the training councils which now have no legislative link and no longer share administration and premises.

The early years of the health visitor council were spent in designing a new syllabus and helping existing training schools to implement it. This took some three years and by 1965 a new educational system was in being. This involved major changes in philosophy and administration for many schools. Prior to 1965 training centres were organised largely on an *ad hoc* basis by local authorities, in addition to some which were sited in Universities and Colleges of Further Education or run by independent bodies such as the RCN and

QAIDNS. A mandatory national examination was organised by the Royal Society of Health, an authorisation granted in 1925 by the then Ministry of Health. All training centres had to submit students for this national assessment before they could practise health visiting in the United Kingdom.

The CETHV abolished the national examination and vested the responsibility for assessment of students in each training centre. Successful candidates were then awarded the Health Visiting Certificate of the CETHV and thus qualified to practise as health visitors. A number of new training schools were established in Colleges of Further Education and Universities and gradually all those not in the mainstream of general education transferred their training centres into colleges. In 1977 there are some 47 training schools in the UK, 9 in Universities and 38 in Polytechnics and Colleges of Further Education. Each school is associated with a catchment area for practical work and has a formal link with health authorities over fieldwork training for its students. The Council agrees the curriculum and examination system for schools on an individual basis and has links with external examiners appointed. Each school also has a Council professional adviser to consult when necessary and this officer acts as liaison between College or University and CETHV. Students are indexed by the Council when they start the course and receive the CETHV certificate at the end if successful in the theoretical and practical assessments of the educational institution. In 1975/6, 1,435 health visitors were trained in this way.

Students are seconded by Area Health Authorities for the course and have to contract to serve in the National Health Service for two years after the course is completed. Where possible this service should be immediately as a health visitor in order to consolidate the professional skills which have been taught.

So much for the main organisational aspect of health visitor training. We should now consider its content and methods of teaching, and also the various types of courses available.

In preparing the syllabus the CETHV had regard to the skills required by the potential health visitor and also the content of her previous training in nursing and midwifery. Objectives in training are based on the view that the work of the health visitor has five main aspects.

(a) the prevention of mental, physical and emotional ill health or the alleviation of its consequences

(b) early detection of ill health and the surveillance of high risk groups
(c) recognition and identification of need and mobilisation of appropriate resources where necessary
(d) health teaching
(e) provision of care; this would include support during periods of stress, and advice and guidance in cases of illness as well as in the care and management of children.[4]

The course must therefore help students to reach the following goals:

(a) to develop that skill in establishing inter-personal relationships which will provide a basis for constructive work with families and individuals
(b) to sharpen the student's perception of early deviation from the normal
(c) to give a knowledge of various statutory and voluntary agencies which may assist in any particular family situation
(d) to provide practice in working out, with families or individuals, programmes of help where these are required and
(e) to illustrate and practise methods of health education and to help develop a critical attitude in their use.

The education required built on the previous professional training as a general nurse with at least three months obstetric training and possibly three months secondment for psychiatry. It is fair to assume, therefore, that entrants into health visiting have basic professional knowledge of physiology and pathological processes and considerable observational skills. All these are necessary if they are to practise effectively as health visitors. They are particularly so in the contemporary work setting which brings the health visitor of the seventies into close contact with the sick and handicapped as well as with the healthy.

    This last situation obtains through the increasing association with general medical practice which has arisen with the growth of primary health care teams. The old style organisation of the health visitor's work on a basis of geographical district responsibility has given place to a variety of links with family doctors, all of which are based on the principle that the health visitor's family caseload coincides with the patients on a doctor's list. This enables the health visitor to have access to all age groups in need of health education and social advice, and aims to bring doctor and health visitor together for reciprocal referrals of individuals who may be in need of either worker's particular expertise. If the health visitor is to carry out the 'prime role' identified by Jameson it is necessary for the Primary Health Care team to have within it other nursing staff who concentrate on the clinical curative aspects of the practice, and social work staff who can take on the work for which they are specially trained. In this context prevention, to the health visitor, embraces the concepts described by Caplan,[5] namely primary prevention based on positive health teaching, secondary prevention based on teaching to avoid relapse into ill-health, and tertiary prevention to assist the handicapped or the aged to live as full a life as possible within the limits of their disabilities. Often the latter type of prevention involves working with colleagues and, for the health visitor, an extensive knowledge of the social sources for reference as well as the skills of effective referral itself.

At the beginning of this paper reference was made to the health visitor as part of the nursing team and this must not be forgotten. In her role as health counsellor and teacher she extends the nursing process and, in a different way, uses similar professional skills to her nursing colleagues. Her assessment of need for nursing care is allied to social diagnosis as much as to medical diagnosis, her plan for her client or patient must be made in concert with other community workers but most of all with the client himself and his family. It involves the support, counselling and positive teaching that she is able to provide from her own store of knowledge as well as referral to others for their expertise. In particular the former centres on child health care and development, family nutrition and budgeting and general interpretation of much that is in the medical field and in the social services. Health and medicine always include mental and emotional aspects as well as physical. Referral to others often involves her skills in interpersonal relations where clients need active persuasion to seek help for incipient problems, or resist the need to involve additional and often unknown workers in their problems. In all this the health visitor is well placed to initiate action as she is the only worker with regular access to normal families for the purpose of health surveillance before breakdown occurs and therefore her visits are not associated in the client's mind with guilt on account of failure to conform with society's expectations and requirements. Unfortunately the current staffing of the service is such that much surveillance of healthy families has had to give place to 'crisis' visiting, much of which is really the province of over-pressed social workers, who are equally short of trained personnel. Association with general medical practice has also increased their load of work with aged, sick and handicapped to the detriment of work with children. This is well recognised by health visitors themselves and has been highlighted in the recently published report of the Court Committee[6] with its recommendation that specialised 'child health visitors' should be appointed. (In reality these would be better named 'family health visitors' as the need to operate within the context of family and extended family is paramount if children's health and development physically, educationally, emotionally and socially are to be safeguarded.)

To achieve all this the CETHV devised an educational programme for pending health visitors which was organised in educational establishments where they could work alongside other students and often share teaching with them. The orthodox course lasts a calendar year and consists of theoretical teaching and fieldwork practice in approximately equal proportion. The first nine months period is based on the college and during this time the theoretical syllabus is covered by lectures, seminars and tutorial work. There is concurrent fieldwork during which students are attached to fieldwork teachers on an individual basis and are taught the practical skills of health visiting. Close linkage between fieldwork teacher and course tutor assist with the application of theory to practice. Both tutors and fieldwork teachers are trained for their tasks, the tutors through a year's course in professional educational method applied to health visiting and the fieldwork teachers over a six-week period especially geared to the imparting of professional skills. CETHV maintains a roll of tutors and issues letters of recognition to fieldwork teachers, thus maintaining more than a watching brief over the qualifications of staff involved in teaching health visitor students.

At the end of the academic year students take their theoretical examinations and then spend three months continuous health visiting practice under special supervision of field and management health visiting staff. They are each made responsible for a small caseload of about 100 families. This is about one fifth of the recommended caseload for health visitors. They learn how to organise their work and gain experience in achieving a balance in priorities. As the health visitor is recognised as an independent worker (and was so described in the Briggs report on nursing in 1972)[7] this is an important proficiency. The final assessment hurdle comes at the end of the course. Students, during the concurrent fieldwork while at college and under supervision of their tutors and fieldwork teachers, visit and study in

depth a very small number of families. These are selected to typify
the preventive and supportive care elements of the health visitor's work.
Health visiting students are presented for examination, together with
an analytical study of the neighbourhood in which the student undertook
her practical work. An oral examination is conducted by internal and
external examiners and is based on the material contained in these
studies. By this means it is possible to assess the students' understanding
of their work in a broad context. Students must pass the theoretical
examination and the oral before qualifying for the CETHV's Certificate
to practise health visiting.

The actual content of the syllabus has been left until last because,
to understand its relevance, it was thought necessary to discuss its aims
and method of implementation. The coverage concerns knowledge
and skills related to the needs of a health teacher to understand
her clientele and also to possess the necessary information to impart.
There are five sections to the syllabus, the first is headed 'Development
of the Individual' and concerns the psychological, physiological and
educational characteristics of individuals from childhood to old age.
Inherent in this section are the environmental and personal factors
required for average healthy development and some discussion of
states of handicap and their origins. The second section is sociological
and is entitled 'The Individual in the Group'. Norms of society are
considered and special attention given to the social institutions relevant
to health visiting practice. Of particular interest is the family and the
school. So too is the position of women and special groups such
as immigrants. This section is particularly relevant when the health
visitor engages on any plan of health education.

The third section is entitled 'Development of Social Policy' and it is
this one which assists in the understanding of the present administrative
structure of the health and social services by putting it in the developmental context of past policies.

Fourthly, the medical and epidemiological knowledge is covered
in a section called 'Social Aspects of Health and Disease' and the
fifth section is the one which spills over from theory into practice
in that it is concerned with the skills of health visiting. It is entitled
'Principles and Practice of Health Visiting' and covers the theory of
health education for groups and individuals, of constructive listening
and associated communication skills and also the organisational
activities which the health visitor needs if she is to handle a caseload
effectively and relate well to professional colleagues and managers.

As well as the orthodox one year course for SRNs, there are a number of other routes to health visiting. These have developed during the last 20 years as experimental schemes. The so-called 'integrated courses' combined nursing, obstetric and health visitor curricula to shorten and co-ordinate teaching for school leavers who wished, from the onset of their career, to enter health visiting. These courses were designed for candidates of university entrance standard at a time when degree programmes for nurses were unknown in the United Kingdom. They are gradually being phased out as broader-based nursing degree courses are established. Currently there is one integrated course of sub-degree standard which is still admitting students. This is at Croydon College of Design and Technology and is associated with King's College Hospital for nurse training. Two degree courses include the health visiting qualification as well as the SRN. One is Manchester University Bachelor of Nursing degree and the other is a sandwich course organised at Southampton University with St Thomas' Hospital. This is a Social Sciences honours degree in the School of Sociology and Social Administration and the structure of the degree provides coverage for the Psychology, Sociology and Social Policy context of the health visitor syllabus while the presence of a long established one year health visitor course in the Sociology Department provides the professional teaching in Social Medicine and health visiting. The new medical school of the University is involved in the medical aspects. The link with St Thomas' Hospital will be phased out after the intake of students in 1977/8 as the hospital is now linked to the Polytechnic of the South Bank for nursing degree studies. When the break occurs the University will continue to offer its degree with health visitor option (without the hospital nursing sandwich) to already qualified SRNs who wish to combine a degree in Social Sciences with health visiting. This programme can be completed in 3 calendar years and has already been successfully followed over the past few years by SRN candidates.

Also in higher education there are opportunities for post-graduate health visitor course study in modified courses in several universities and polytechnics engaged in CNAA degree work for nurses. These are relatively new ventures but will probably develop further as the post-graduate need becomes more widespread.

This then is an account of health visiting as we know it today, and the current educational preparation for the work. To describe the job effectively is difficult; this paper has therefore not attempted to do this, but has merely set out to provide some information to assist those who are interested in understanding what a health visitor aims to do and how she is educated to achieve her goals.

Notes

1. National Health Service Act (1946), Sec. 24 and 28.
2. *An Inquiry into Health Visiting*, report of a Working Party on the field of work, training and recruitment of health visitors (HMSO, London, 1956).
3. Report of the Working Party on social workers in the local authority health and welfare services. (HMSO, London, 1959).
4. Council for the Education and Training of Health Visitors, *The Function of the Health Visitor* (CTHV, London, 1967).
5. G. Caplan, *An Approach to Community Mental Health* (Tavistock, London, 1967).
6. *Fit for the Future,* the Report of the Committee on Child Health Services (HMSO, London, 1977).
7. Report of the Committee on Nursing (Cmnd 5150, HMSO, London, 1972).

7 PRODUCERS AND CONSUMERS – A VIEW OF COMMUNITY HEALTH COUNCILS

Pat Gordon

In their short lives community health councils have aroused a lot of strong feelings. Many people who know more or less about it, have felt moved to express their opinions. Reference to watchdogs and teeth are perhaps the most common but there are many others. David Owen, for example, has written: 'The decision to establish community health councils will probably be looked back on by social historians as the most significant aspect of the whole NHS reorganisation. . .' *Which?* magazine: 'CHCs should be an important new voice for the consumer in the NHS.' *The Times*: 'Public watchdogs ready to influence service.' Wandsworth & East Merton CHC: 'snivelling lapdogs or rabid curs?' NHS administrator: 'no facts, only gut reactions.' SRN in *Nursing Mirror*: 'Is it too much to ask for an end to the fault finding which so many members of CHCs seem to think is their only function?' Chairman, Local Dental Committee: 'Most people on my side of the fence see CHCs as a bloody nuisance.'

There has been much generalisation but little detail. This paper will try to describe some of the facts about CHCs, their activities and achievements, and leave the reader to judge for himself whether to see them as 'the most significant aspect of reorganisation' or 'a bloody nuisance.' In making his decision, he would do well to consider two fundamental questions. First, what is health? If he sees health as a commodity produced by the NHS and consumed by the public, this will give him one perspective. If on the other hand, he sees health as something very much more than that, something which we each have power to influence and take responsibility for, then his perspective will change. Margaret Stacey has developed the argument that if we see ourselves as consumers of services provided by the NHS, we relegate ourselves to a passive rather than an active role.[1] If we see ourselves as active producers of health and ill-health, our view of the world and how we might influence it will change.

The second question is, who is the NHS organised for? Health workers would answer that the NHS is organised to meet the public's needs and most of them work long, hard hours to achieve this. Yet large sections of the public know that their needs are not being met, despite the hard work and the vast expenditure of money.

If services do not meet needs, the next questions must be how do we define need and how do we assess whether services are doing what we think they are? These kinds of questions generate long debate which is not appropriate here but it is within the experience of all of us to know, as Wandsworth & East Merton CHC have said, that the health service planner brought up in a hospital-based medical service will have a different concept of needs from the Wandsworth pensioner whose main concern is to stay out of hospital 'because hospitals are where you go to die.'[2] Community health councils have a part to play in reconciling these different views and getting the balance right.

CHCs are not a new species. The 'consumer' has a long history in running the NHS. As an elected member of local government, he played a large part in providing and monitoring what are now known as community health services. As The Layman, he was a member of Hospital Management Committees and Regional Hospital Boards, part manager, part employer, part consumer representative. Some worked wonders, but the prevailing attitude seems to have been of deference to the experts. The novelty about CHCs was that for the first time the consumer was to be independent. He would have no part in managing, employing or providing services. Jean Robinson of the Patients' Association describes an incident which illustrates this. In Oxfordshire recently, health authority administrators were asked to come to a CHC meeting to put their case for the closure of a local hospital. They were questioned for over an hour. She goes on, 'I never as a regional hospital board member saw people put through the mill as those were. Yet on the regional hospital board the officials were our employees. . . The attitude was that the officials were the experts and must know best.'[3]

Laymen have been involved in other ways too. Ethical Committees have a statutory layman. Perhaps one of the best examples of this kind were the committees formed in the early 1960s to decide who should get kidney machines. There are Patients' Committees such as the one attached to the Aberdare Health Centre which started by complaining about the appointments system and the doctors' rota and gradually moved on to study-sessions on breast cancer, abortion, euthanasia and screening for the over-60s. The Patients' Association is well known and its reputation rests perhaps on its determination not to be browbeaten by professionals. They have made it their business to be well-informed and have not retreated from arguments on clinical issues. When CHCs were formed, it is said the Patients' Association considered bowing out, its task over. This has not happened and its task is clearly not over yet.

CHCs were an afterthought. When Sir Keith Joseph employed McKinsey to reorganise the NHS, his overriding aim was to have good management. The final solution was to appoint Regional Health Authorities who would appoint Area Health Authorities who would appoint District Management Teams, who would then manage the whole thing efficiently from top to bottom. The NHS Reorganisation Bill was well on its way through the legislative process before CHCs came into it. In its passage through the House of Lords, there were so many protests about its undemocratic nature that the idea of community health councils was introduced. Each district was to have its own health council, separate from management, whose job would be to represent to managers the views of the people. The original proposals were that health councils would live in premises provided by their area health authority, run their affairs on money provided by their area health authority and take as their secretaries bright young managers on their way up the NHS ladder who could be spared for a year or two, or bright old managers who had given a lifetime's service to the NHS and knew the system so well they could service two or three councils before retirement. The beginnings were not auspicious. No wonder the toothless watchdog appeared.

However, several things happened which have gone a long way to changing that. The government changed three weeks before reorganisation was to take place. The new Secretary of State introduced a paper called 'Democracy in the Health Service' which was to strengthen CHCs in two important ways.[4] They were to be free to appoint their own secretaries by open competition. Bright young managers were no longer obligatory. This has brought to the NHS people from all sorts of disciplines with varying perceptions, attitudes and skills and has been a positive benefit. Secondly, CHCs were given powers over hospital closures. If an Area Health Authority proposed closing a hospital or changing its use and the CHC agreed, they could go ahead. If the CHC opposed closure and produced well-argued alternative proposals and there was still no agreement, the decision would have to be passed upwards to the Region and the Minister. The important factor which has come out of this is not the number of closures which the Minister has approved despite CHC opposition, but the number of proposals which have been reconsidered, modified or completely overturned at Area and Regional level as a result of CHC intervention. In these cases the Minister is not involved but the end result has been achieved of giving the local community a strong voice in what happens to its hospitals.

Another thing which happened after reorganisation was that far
more people were interested in the idea of a local health council
than anyone had imagined. In Haringey in North London, for example,
200 voluntary organisations wanted to make nominations for the dozen
seats available to them on the CHC.

When CHCs were set up in 1974 there were very few rules about
what they should do, possibly because no-one had time to think them up.
This has allowed individual CHCs to develop in very different ways in
response to different pressures and different interests and energies.
There were, however, certain guidelines. CHCs were to try to provide
information to the public, to comment on how local health services
work, to visit hospitals and clinics and comment on what they saw, to
provide information to health authorities and to help people with
complaints. Three of these guidelines will be looked at here and used
to illustrate what CHCs have done.

Information to the Public

Some people saw this as little more than a means of using CHCs as a
cheap PRO for the health service. If cuts were to be imposed and
unwelcome decisions made, CHCs could be used to convince the public
of their necessity. This may have happened in some places, but
certainly not in all.

CHCs have interpreted their task of giving information to the public
in many ways. One way is to write it down. City & Hackney CHC has
recently published a people's guide to the health service entitled
'Health in Hackney — The NHS and how to make it work for you.'[5]
The idea is to tell people about their local health services and
encourage them to use them to advantage. There are general sections
about hospitals and chemists and ambulances and so on and other
sections for people who use the NHS more than most, like mothers with
small children and elderly people. It explains how to get hospital
treatment, second opinions, change doctors, mend spectacles, complain
to the Ombudsman, avoid unexpected dental bills and protest about
unsafe conditions at work. It also tries to encourage people to take
more responsibility for their treatment and not to be frightened of
asking questions.

The guide explains how the system *should* work but it also
acknowledges that advising people to 'go to your family doctor' or 'go
to your social service office' does not always get them very far. So there
are names and addresses of other people and organisations in the

neighbourhood who know what's going on and can help.

The NHS is not noted for its easy, open literature or its ability to publicise services and encourage people to use them well. The guide book is an attempt by the CHC to fill that gap on the grounds that if the consumer is to play a responsible part in deciding the kind of health service we have, the more we know and understand the better.

It is often said that people are not interested in the health service until they are ill but when the City & East London Area Health Authority proposed radically reorganising hospital services in Hackney more than 500 people came to the CHC's meeting to hear these proposals. It was the largest public meeting in the district for years. Before 1974 proposals such as these were made by Hospital Management Committees and Regional Boards, and who ever knew what they were planning?

Some time after this meeting, when the proposals had been drastically altered, we learned we were to get a 'nucleus' hospital. Such were the murmurs and confusion about atomic medicine and nuclear hospitals that the CHC asked the DHSS to come to the district and explain what a nucleus hospital was. Over 100 people came to hear them.

There are other ways of telling people what's going on. Some CHCs have shopfronts. In Kent and in Leeds they have regular programmes on local radio. In Kensington one of the CHCs produced a newspaper which was distributed to every household. In Lambeth in central London, St Thomas's CHC has its own shop. Local kids used to wander in after school and ask if there was anything for them to do. This led the CHC to question how they could make real contact with these children. This in turn led to a health event in the Easter holidays where 30 local children learnt about diet and nutrition. It sounds very worthy and earnest, but it wasn't at all like that. The CHC wanted to make the children think about what makes health. They decided to concentrate on food and digestion and to use wholemeal bread as the weapon. They visited the local baker and watched him bake brown bread. They listened to Dr Stanway who wrote the book *Taking the rough with the smooth*. They baked wholemeal bread in the kitchens at the back of the CHC shop. It was all enormous fun, and much more. Several children have been back to say they or their mothers have baked brown bread for the first time; two boys bought apples instead of sweets with their pocket money; most of the children have stopped bringing sweets into the CHC shop. One mother came in to say that for the first time ever her daughter had voluntarily eaten greens 'because

the doctor at the health council said it was good for her.' A weekly
health club has been set up and when the children were recently
asked 'what is health?' several included things like eating properly,
being happy, cleaning your teeth. This compares with earlier
discussions when they could all give long lists of diseases under the
heading Illness, but precious little under Health.[6]

This kind of information is commonly known as health education,
but not in the style of moral exhortation which we can all now
recognise and ignore. Small-scale projects which are local and
relevant are the CHC's strength. Along the same lines are the
Wandsworth CHC's meetings on health issues, bringing information
and opinion to people to help them decide for themselves. When
they had an evening meeting on birth, with a film on home
confinements and one on Leboyer's methods, the hall was full with
standing room only. And afterwards there was a chance to discuss
the issues with local doctors and midwives.

Information to Health Authorities

Information to health authorities was to be another task CHCs were to
attempt. For some people this meant that CHCs would do little more
than reflect emotional outcries at hospital closures or impossible and
ill-informed demands for more and better services. This too may have
happened in some places but certainly not in all.

Services for the elderly are more and more recognised as one of
the most inadequate and badly needed of our health services. In
Worthing the elderly population is 27 per cent of the total, one of the
highest in the country. If you live in Worthing you know how hard it is
to get an old person into hospital. Relatives are often left with the
choice of a nursing home, and the expense that entails, or nursing the
ill person themselves at home. The CHC in Worthing decided they had
to find out what the need for community care was and how far the
services provided were meeting that need. This I think is the most
useful and potentially the most powerful thing CHCs can do, choose
some aspect of the NHS in their neighbourhood and find out whether
it really works the way it is said to.

The impressive thing about the Worthing project is that they
recognised that to be of any value it had to be a reliable survey. They
knew they did not have the resources to do it themselves yet they
did not want it to go to an outside body over whose policy they would
have no control. The solution was to use the Government's Job
Creation Scheme and with guidance from local doctors and the

university they employed six interviewers and interviewed more than 2,000 elderly people. Instead of just complaining about inadequate services, instead of just echoing the health authority which acknowledged that there was 'a problem', they went out and researched it and wrote a booklet which describes what it is like to be an old person living in Worthing.[7]

They have achieved stage one of the battle by providing the health authority with detailed information about their neighbourhood. The second stage, which they are now well into, is to persuade them to act on it. Here too they seem to be succeeding, however slowly. Discussions are under way with dentists and opticians about getting information to old people, about joint funding of health and social service projects, and the district managers, with one of the highest percentages of old people in the country, have at last set up a working party on their needs.

Another example of this kind of information gathering which is small-scale and local and relevant is the study planned by Wandsworth and East Merton CHC with their local Community Relations Council. There is a large Asian community in their neighbourhood and they want to find out why there is such a poor uptake of community health services by Asian women and children.

CHC can come up with information in other ways too. During the time of the James White Abortion Amendment Bill, many CHCs discussed the issues and came to their various conclusions. In Hackney the CHC decided to try to find out how the Abortion Act was working in the district. We wrote to the district managers and to the obstetricians and gynaecologists to ask for factual information. The obstetricians did not reply. The district administrator said he had no information and no means of getting it and felt that we should accept that 'terminations of pregnancy are provided within the constraints of available resources within this District in accordance with the laws made by Parliament.'

David Owen, when he was Minister of Health, constantly reminded us that access to information is power in a democracy and he upbraided administrators who criticised CHCs for uninformed criticism and at the same time denied them the information on which to base informed criticism. We might add that if administrators do not have information and can see no way of getting it, CHCs can sometimes help. In this case, we got information from the Registrar General's Statistical Review, from the Hospital Activity Analysis, from the British Pregnancy Advisory Service. We talked to local

women, health visitors, doctors and social workers. We built up a
picture of the service in our district and when we published the report
it caused a considerable stir. Among other things it showed that in
1973 (the latest available figures at the time) only 35 per cent of
Hackney women who had an abortion had it on the NHS. There was
strong support from local GPs for an improved service. The
obstetricians disputed the figures. The Area Health Authority
acknowledged the inadequate service and undertook a review of
abortion services across the whole area. Now a year later, a day care
unit has been established in one part of the area where sympathetic
doctors have long been fighting for it. The quibble over statistics still
goes on but what is important is that by not giving up, by digging
around for officially published data and putting it together so that
its local relevance became clear, the CHC has supplied information
and pressure for change which would otherwise have been missing.

CHCs often feel that they are the only ones to question the
assumptions of health service planners and to question the data, or
the lack of data, on which plans are based. But as well as *asking* for
facts and figures, it is clear that some CHCs have already contributed
a great deal to the information available on health needs and health
services.

Complaints

My third example of the guidelines for CHCs concerns complaints.
CHCs were given the task of helping people who have a complaint
about the NHS, but not of investigating that complaint. For many
professionals, this was the last straw. And it is disheartening even now
to talk to doctors, especially GPs, and to nurses who say 'So you're
the ones out to make trouble.' The only conclusion I fear is that the
medical press must have published some really hair-raising articles
about the advent of CHCs, and attitudes change only slowly. In fact,
there have been no long queues of people marching to their CHC to
complain about their doctor. Nor have CHCs gone into the market
place to ferment revolt.

What has happened is that, rather than complaints, CHCs have had
far more requests for information and help from people trying to find
their way around the health and social services obstacle course.
Secondly, although the 'gratitude barrier' has not been broken and
people have not suddenly become eager to complain, CHCs have found
themselves listening to grumbles and confusion and criticism and
anxieties about things which have gone wrong. They have built up a

picture of the NHS in action, previously known only to those who run
the service, or perhaps not even to them. Liverpool Central and
Southern CHC has recently published a booklet which they call 'A
Profile of Patients' Problems' in which they analyse the 300 complaints
and requests for help they received in 1976.[8]

> In our experience very few people are malicious or vindictive or wish
> for a financial settlement. Most often they want proper investigation
> into their problem, an acknowledgment from the Health Service that
> procedure could be improved and evidence that steps could be
> taken to ensure as far as possible that what has happened to them will
> not happen to other people. . .In the main, people do not want to
> see themselves as complainants. Often they had to be given
> reassurance that they were not being unreasonable. Guilt about
> complaining bracketed with low expectations of the service, lack
> of information and a fear of victimisation, militate against easy
> public expression of dissatisfaction.

I think most CHCs would echo that, although there are outspoken
members of the medical profession and their defence societies who
would dispute it.

In the last year the DHSS has asked for comments on whether to
change three different aspects of the complicated complaints
procedures. CHCs have given their evidence along with others and this
has brought a valuable perspective which would otherwise have been
missing.

As well as helping individuals through the complaints procedures,
the CHC can take up general issues from specific complaints. In our
district, we seemed to get a spate of complaints about longer and
longer delays in chiropody appointments. We raised it with the
district managers and then with the Area Health Authority. It was not
clear whether this was happening throughout the area or whether it
was peculiar to our neighbourhood. The Authority commissioned a
survey which showed, among other things, that in our district fewer
patients were treated than in the other two districts and the cost per
patient per year was three times as high. A number of very practical
recommendations were made and the whole position is to be reviewed
again in the autumn.

In Cheshire, the Halton CHC found that many of the complaints
they received related to receptionists. They decided to set up a
meeting between the CHC and the receptionists. Out of 18 practices

in the district, they got 21 receptionists and from the start it was clear
that they cared a great deal about the service they gave and what the
public thought of it. What was even more interesting as the discussion
went on was that very few receptionists were given training of any
kind. Most of them developed their ideas of the job in terms of
protecting the doctor from the patients. Few were ever included in
policy discussions in their practice. Only two had ever seen how
another practice was run and all of them were meeting together for the
first time. And yet as everyone knows, the receptionist can be a
crucial part of a visit to a GP or a health centre. Following the CHC
initiative, some of the receptionists now meet together to exchange
ideas about the NHS and their role in it. And Halton CHC has joined
with South Tyneside CHC and almost 100 others in urging the DHSS
to take steps to provide more training for receptionists. The DHSS
has taken it up and a report is on its way. One of the problems
however is bound to be that GPs are independent contractors and
health authorities have very little influence over how they run their
practices.

None of the above is meant to imply that CHCs have an exclusive
claim on what the consumer thinks about the health service. Many
doctors and administrators and other producers of services know
only too well what is needed and fight very hard to get it. What is
clear is that CHCs have demonstrated that their perspective is very
important in getting the balance right. There are many other
examples that could be used — marvellous commonsense things like
Tower Hamlets CHC pressing for the psychogeriatric ward to be
moved from the top floor to the bottom; Leeds CHCs discovering
there was only one centre in the city to which people had to travel
to get batteries for their hearing aids. Now batteries are available at
centres all over the city. Some CHCs have produced influential
work on the health needs of decaying inner cities. Some have had a
lot to say about health needs in districts in the hinterland of teaching
hospitals. Some have started to take up the biggest challenge, that
of the professional expert.

There are 229 health councils in England and Wales and 40 in
Scotland. They vary enormously. It is a comfort to know that
professionals vary too. Recently I met a very senior nurse who said she
thought her local CHC was 'a bunch of middle class communists.' Three
days later I met a doctor who said he thought CHCs were the best
possible allies in getting a rational health service. Perhaps there will
always be strong opinions, and perhaps that is no bad thing.

Notes

1. *CHC News*, No.7, May 1976 (Wandsworth & East Merton CHC Annual Report, 1976).
2. Wandsworth & East Merton CHC Annual Report, 1976 (1 Balham Station Road, SW12).
3. Jean Robinson, *The Times*, 11 February 1976.
4. 'Democracy in the Health Service' (HMSO, London, 1974).
5. 'Health in Hackney – the NHS and how to make it work for you' (City & Hackney Hackney CHC, 210 Kingsland Road, E2 8EB).
6. Sally Weston and Susan Thorne, 'CHC bakes a health cake' in *CHC News*, No.22 (August 1977).
7. 'Concern for the Elderly' (Worthing CHC, 1 Victoria Buildings, York Road, Worthing, 1977).
8. 'A Profile of Patients' Problems' (Liverpool Central & Southern CHC, 80 Rodney Street, Liverpool L1 9AP).

8 THE CONTROL OF TECHNOLOGY IN THE INTERESTS OF HEALTH

Ernest Braun

If the importance of a topic were measured by the number of
ways in which its title can be interpreted, then there could be no
doubt that we are dealing with a topic of major importance. For
we could interpret the title of this talk in numerous ways and,
to do it full justice, should deal with it in all these ways. We should
discuss first the control of technology in general and then perhaps
the very concept of health. This latter is a task so difficult
that it will have to be relegated to the ranks of the many things
that space will not permit us to tackle here. The list of such
topics is long: the control of technology to ensure safety
at work, road safety, safety of domestic appliances and the
home generally. The whole area of medical engineering,
including the allocation of resources for x-ray machines, kidney
machines, and all the rest of modern medical machinery.
Equally it would be interesting but not practicable in this context
to consider the control of the development and use of drugs.
Finally, we could talk about all aspects of environmental control,
starting with sanitation and ending with the ozone layer. We shall
not attempt to examine all this, but will select some small segments
from this vast area.

Indeed, this paper is confined to a few general remarks about the
control of technology for the public good and to a few remarks
about making decisions on environmental controls in the face of
considerable scientific uncertainty about the effects of some
pollutants.

Technology, like most activities in our kind of society, is
controlled by a complex web of interlinked mechanisms. The main
ingredients of the control system are market forces, legislation
and incentives. We could enter a deep political debate as to which
of these ingredients should predominate, but it is not difficult to
achieve a broad consensus that all three are necessary.

The market mechanism operates mainly in two ways in our field
of interest: to promote new products which can be sold to the
health services or the public, e.g. disposable syringes, surgical tools,

drugs, water purifiers and many more. Often, the market mechanism is stimulated and aided by research and development effort paid for by the public. The second way in which the free market operates is in the prevention of pollution and other damage if, and only if, it is more economic not to pollute or damage.

Compounds will not be discharged from a factory, on purely economic grounds, if it is cheaper to retain and re-use them. One might argue that very obviously harmful devices will not be brought on the market because nobody would buy them, but this argument requires a degree of faith in human wisdom which I, for one, find difficult to sustain.

The free market mechanism obviously plays a major role in the control of much of the technology we use, but as far as the control of technology in the interest of health is concerned, the market operates to a limited extent only and no advanced society places much faith in it.

Market forces can be made to operate more to public advantage by a variety of incentives and disincentives. At the simplest level, the imposition of fines on polluters may be regarded as an economic disincentive to cause pollution. On a somewhat more sophisticated level, the provision of research laboratories, research grants, university courses on environmental health and the control of pollution, public analyst laboratories, and all the rest of the government-supported infra-structure requisite for the effective control of health hazards may be regarded as providing positive incentives. Into this category fall direct grants for research into harmful effects of some chemicals or radiation or whatever, but also grants for the development of new medical machinery. So interwoven is the structure of knowledge and of technology, that any advance in knowledge may lead to an invention of a new medically useful process or the control of a medically harmful effect. The whole government structure of open laboratories, and generally the research support system, may be viewed as incentives to the promotion of health by science and technology. Although indirect incentives are important, they are far outweighed by direct support for positive measures. Indeed government supported research and development activities, government supported advisory committees, government purchasing power, and government supported health education in the broadest sense; all these form the major tier of control of technology by positive incentives.

From positive incentives to do medically useful things, to negative incentives in the sense of disincentives to do medically harmful things. Apart from legislation, which we shall speak of separately, there is the incentive of maintaining a good public image. This is particularly strong in the United States, where public opinion is strongly aligned behind the environmental lobby. Even in the United Kingdom, it is important to firms to be seen to be public-spirited, to have the health and safety of citizens and workers at heart. I do believe that this motivation is real and important and that the public could make it even more important. Perhaps it is a mistake to call this kind of motivation a disincentive to do harm, perhaps we should view it rather as a positive incentive, a positive will, to do good.

Some economists of repute have advocated the introduction of pricing of the use of the environment in an attempt to minimize the use of legislation and maximize the use of financial incentives and thereby to extend the operation of market forces. Financial incentives would be such as to transfer the use of the environment into the sphere of market economics. A manufacturer could purchase the right to pollute a river or the air. If the price were right, so the argument goes, pollution would be kept within any desired limits. It seems to me that the belief in pricing environmental pollution is based on a blind and doctrinaire faith in the boundless wisdom of the market economy. For surely to price pollution it must be detected and measured and acceptable limits must be set. Thus a public involvement becomes necessary, inspectors must be appointed, standards set investigated. If this is so, then the simplest, cheapest and most honest method of enforcing the standards is by legislation, rather than by some artificial pricing mechanism. The public, or the government on its behalf, cannot escape the duty of setting up regulations which control the use of technology in the interest of safety and health. Whether it be regulations about the safety of machinery, or the design of motor vehicles, or the use of drugs or x-ray machines, or environmental pollution; the need for regulation is inescapable.

To deal with gross and obvious pollution is relatively easy. We have been successful in eliminating many infectious diseases by suitable sanitation and by the provision of pure water. We have reduced the incidence of some bronchial disorders by the clean air acts. We have made some progress in the cleaning of foul waterways. The really difficult problems are those where there is considerable scientific uncertainty.

We know that the incidence of certain diseases has increased

manyfold in recent years. We know that our environment — the food
we eat, the water we drink, the air we breathe — contains many
chemicals which may, singly or in combination, cause disease. We do
not know, however, what quantities, what combinations, what
compounds are harmful or the extent of their harm. Should we suspect
environmental pollution as the cause of some diseases of civilisation?
How can we find out?

Other papers in this collection by my colleagues will deal with two
specific aspects of these general questions; one with the experimental
screening of compounds for carcinogens, the other with policies for
the control of environmental pollution by heavy metals. A few
comments on the general problem of decisions in the face of
uncertainty may however be made here.

Let us take the example of lead and cadmium. No doubt, the
ingestion of large doses of these metals causes acute poisoning. The
substances are toxic beyond dispute. But what, if any, effect do
small quantities absorbed over a long period of time have? How small
need the quantities be before their effect becomes negligible or
even beneficial? How do these metals interact with other environmental
factors in their toxicity? Are all individuals equally at risk when they
are exposed to the same concentrations of these metals in air or water
or food or cigarettes? Our answers to these questions are uncertain.
We searched the scientific literature for an unequivocal answer. We
found much material, many papers, articles and books — but no
unequivocal answer. Many authors assert with assurance the
establishment of certain facts about the damage caused by very small
doses of this or that metal. Equally many authors assert with equal
assurance the lack of causal links or even correlation between
exposure and damage.

It has been argued, for example, that cadmium in water causes
hypertension and heart disease. It has been argued also that lead
ingested by children causes hyperactivity, lack of concentration and
behavioural problems. It has also been argued that there is no
conclusive evidence to substantiate these and many other suspicions.

To the layman and scientist alike this situation is not only
frustrating, but also most surprising. One sits back and says to oneself
that, when all is said and done, it should be possible to devise a few
good experiments to establish the truth of the matter. But the
difficulties are formidable as can be appreciated by brief references to
a few of them. First, there is the difficulty of detection and
measurement of very small quantities of metals. Despite considerable

advances in scientific technique, the problem remains formidable. Secondly, there is the problem of knowing how exposure to certain levels of a pollutant is related to the absorption and retention of this pollutant in the body. Even if this difficulty is overcome, it is still difficult to know the metabolic role in different individuals and to understand any mechanisms which might cause damage to the bodily functions. Thirdly, there is the multifactor problem. We are all exposed to a whole array of environmental hazards and, to compound matters, exposure to them is mostly irregular. How are we to find out whether the level of cadmium in water is important only in conjunction with certain eating habits or with the concurrent exposure to some other unknown compound? How are we to know whether environmental exposures incurred many years previously make us more susceptible to some present hazard? Finally, to complete this incomplete tale of woe, we must mention the difficulty of experimental verification. Even if we obtain statistical evidence for a correlation between some environmental factor and the incidence of some disease, we cannot be sure that the correlation uncovers a causal relationship. In a multi-factor situation, the absence of knowledge of cause and effect casts doubt on any correlations and makes their establishment beyond doubt doubly difficult. We obviously cannot experiment with very large numbers of humans under very strictly controlled environmental conditions over a very long period of time. Animal experiments, on the other hand, apart from being objectionable on grounds both of cost and of ethics, tend to be inconclusive in these matters because effects are very specific to specific species. Much of what knowledge we have is therefore obtained from observations on groups of people specifically exposed to a particular hazard, such as workers in a lead smelter. On the other hand, their exposure can be most stringently controlled and, in any case, they do not tend to be representative of the population at large.

No doubt we must continue to investigate these matters. With sufficient ingenuity and sufficient money, probably in that order of importance, it should be possible to continue in the establishment of some facts. Research must go on and its quality must improve all the time. But while we are waiting for new results to confirm our suspicions or allay our fears, we must take the best measures we can to protect ourselves against likely damage.

Clearly, to eliminate all hazards is impossible; but it is perfectly feasible to think of some reasonable ground-rules to deal with a situation of uncertain risks. Let us examine a possible set of such rules:

Rule 1. Assess hazards continuously in the light of the latest
scientific findings.
Rule 2. Reduce the dangers by the most cost-effective methods.
Rule 3. Keep a reasonable balance between safety and economic
or other benefit.
Rule 4. Retain flexibility, so that wrong decisions can be revised.

Not much need be said about our first rule. In an uncertain situation,
we must clearly revise our knowledge continuously and must therefore
revise our estimates of hazards with progressing knowledge. The
question of estimation of hazards is more tricky. If it is impossible to
arrive at numerical estimates, what we must resort to is some
consensus of expert and lay opinion. Perhaps the best hope of
success is if a number of truly independent experts express their views
and these are then judged by some political process. By political
process I mean a process of finding a compromise between the
interests of various groups and finding a balance between extremes of
view.

The second rule requires a little explanation. There are usually many
ways of reducing some known or suspected hazard. If we wish to
reduce the level of cadmium in water, we can forbid the use of
cadmium in all its technical applications and we can discontinue
the use of any water which contains naturally high levels of cadmium.
It may be, however, that the amount of reduction achieved by some
partial prohibition would be almost as great, while the cost might be
a fraction of that of total prohibition. Even the effect of discontinuing
the use of some naturally occurring water rich in cadmium can
be achieved in a different way. It may be cheaper, for example,
to remove the cadmium by some chemical means. Generally speaking,
one must seek various ways of achieving reductions of hazards and
choose the highest reduction at the lowest cost.

What total cost we should incur must, of course, be a matter of
political decision and therefore compromise. It is evident that
to reduce all pollution to zero would mean to cease all activity. Our
third rule must be read in conjunction with our second. A reasonable
balance must be kept between the dangers incurred in some activity
and the benefit obtained from it. A reasonable proportion of the
economic benefit of the activity must be devoted to the reduction,
with greatest possible cost-effectiveness, of the hazards incurred in the

activity. It sounds perfectly plausible; but behind the word reasonable is hidden a whole gamut of political questions. Some of these are easy, some difficult, others totally intractable. The science and politics of the environment are inseparable because they are intertwined precisely in rules such as ours.

This leaves us to discuss our fourth rule. In the face of continual revision of estimates of hazards, it is clearly desirable to retain flexibility of action, so that action can follow knowledge. If we decide to build some plant to remove a certain chemical from our water supply, we must be aware that this plant may soon become obsolete. As far as possible, we should allow for this in design and not sink vast capital resources into what may become a white elephant. Thus when it comes to choosing between greater capital expenditure and greater running costs, we should plunge for greater running costs. Many more examples could be mentioned, but time is short and the one will have to suffice.

This brief review is intended to give some insight into how our society controls technology in the public interest and what special difficulties arise when it comes to the control of some environmental hazards. Hopefully it has also provided at least a little food for thought on how the control processes could be improved.

9 ENVIRONMENTAL CONTROL STRATEGIES FOR LEAD

D. Collingridge, K. Edwards and J. McEvoy

The question of whether levels of lead found in our normal environment are harmful is a highly contentious and much debated one. As we shall see later, much evidence indicating the existence of harm has been brought forward, but none of it is unequivocal and beyond criticism. Any fair review of our existing knowledge about lead must end with the conclusion that we just do not know whether present environmental levels of the metal place anyone at risk. Nevertheless, a decision about whether or not to reduce these levels is unavoidable. If we do nothing, we have at least decided to tolerate existing lead levels. The problem, of course, is how we can make a rational decision where our ignorance is so extensive. Not knowing the extent of the harm possible from environmental levels of lead, we cannot calculate the benefits from reducing these levels, although we can have a good guess at their costs. It is, therefore, impossible to balance the benefits from reducing environmental lead levels with the costs of the reductions.

For this reason, we have attempted to calculate and compare the cost-effectiveness of possible control strategies for environmental lead. The thinking behind this is that if there is a relatively cheap, i.e. highly cost-effective, way of reducing exposure to lead, then, even though we cannot compare the costs involved with the benefits to be derived, we may still decide to adopt the method as an insurance against the possibility that environmental levels of lead are harmful. If, on the other hand, all ways of reducing exposure to lead are very expensive, i.e. have a low cost-effectiveness, then we may decide to save our money and live with the possible dangers from the metal.

In this paper we wish to stress the methodology which we employed in measuring the cost-effectiveness of control strategies for lead. The reason for this is that the methodology seems to be of very general applicability. Our ignorance about lead is really quite typical of our understanding of most pollutants, and weighing benefits from abatement with abatement costs is generally as impossible as it is for lead. Comparison of control strategies for

most pollutants, therefore, calls for a cost-effective approach like the
one we have tried to develop for lead. An important bonus from
using this methodology is that it can indicate what research gaps
exist. Briefly, priority should be given to research whose findings,
one way or the other, are likely to lead to different cost-effective
rankings of the control strategies. If the ranking is likely to be
unaffected by the results of some research, then this research may
be given a low priority.

Work of this kind is obviously interdisciplinary, calling for
contributions from, amongst others, biology, chemistry, chemical
engineering, economics, food technology and systems theory.
Although heavy demands were made on many departments at
Aston and elsewhere, a natural home for this study is provided by
Aston's Technology Policy Unit. The work is continuing, so what
follows is more of a progress report than a finished product.

Firstly the evidence which has been brought forward to show
that environmental levels of lead are harmful will be looked at and
then, in a little more depth, the problem posed by our ignorance on
this score. The methodology adopted will be outlined and each of its
parts considered in detail.

1. Are Environmental Levels of Lead Harmful?

The toxicity of lead was known in antiquity, and the widespread use
of the metal in many industrial processes has provided a substantial
body of knowledge about the harmful effects of continued exposure
to high concentrations. Drawing on experience with industrial lead
workers, Kehoe has suggested that exposure to the metal is harmful
only when it produces blood lead levels above 80 μg/100g of whole blood.[1]
Although cases of lead poisoning associated with lower blood lead
levels have been reported,[2] it seems clear that there is little chance of
an otherwise healthy person suffering the classical symptoms of lead
poisoning from an exposure which produces a blood lead level lower
than Kehoe's limit.

Kehoe's concern was for clinical lead poisoning – poisoning
producing signs or symptoms which are evident to the doctor or
sufferer, such as (for an adult poisoned by inorganic lead) abdominal
pain, constipation, vomiting, general debility and diarrhoea. Whilst
welcoming improvements in industrial hygiene leading to a steady fall
in the number of workers harmed by industrial exposure, many
researchers have expressed fear about a different problem posed by
lead. Evidence is accumulating from a number of quarters that

exposure to low levels of lead, of the sort found in most urban environments, may produce insidious harm, even though the blood levels resulting from the exposure are well below Kehoe's 80 μg/100g limit. Before considering the evidence for this so-called sub-clinical lead poisoning, it must be stressed that none of it is infallible. We still await, and perhaps always will await, proof of the existence of sub-clinical lead poisoning.[3]

The most worrying claims about the sub-clinical effects of lead are that the metal may cause behavioural, mental and developmental disturbances in children who show none of the clinical symptoms of lead poisoning. A study in El Paso, Texas, compared symptomless children with blood lead levels greater than 40 μg/100 ml with children having lower blood levels. Impairment of fine motor, perceptual and visual skills and a lower age-adjusted IQ were found in the high-lead group.[4] Blood lead levels in children near 40 μg/100 ml are common in the US and not unknown in the UK. Figure 9.2, from another study, shows the results from a battery of tests given to 4-year-old children with a high lead exposure, though with no clinical symptoms, and controls.

Figure 9.1: Results of Tests given to 4-Year-old Children with a High Lead Exposure and no Controls

Test	Blood Lead	
	<40 μg/100g	>40 μg/100g
Visual Reaction time[a] (m sec)	26.3	29.2
Auditory Reaction Time[a] (m sec)	24.4	26.1
2-plate Tapping[a] (No. taps)	15.4	15.3
Finger-wrist Tapping[a] (No. taps)	49.8	43.8
Verbal IQ[b]	85.14	83.85
Performance IQ[b]	102.71	94.93
Full-scale IQ[b]	92.88	88.02

Source: Adapted from P. Landrigen *et al.*, *Lancet*, 1 (1975), p.708.

a   Av. of dominant and non-dominant
b   WISC and WPPSI

Figure 9.2: Performance of 4-Year-Olds with Lead Exposure and Controls

Test	Percentage Borderline or Abnormal	
	Lead Exposed Group	Control Group
IQ	24.7	9.8
Fine Motor Area	44.9	25.7
Gross Motor Area	15.9	7.0
Concept Formation	14.7	9.8
Behaviour Profile	30.4	9.7

Source: Adapted from de la Burde *et al.*, *Journal of Pediatrics*, 81 (1972), p.1088.

Studies in the 1960s of blood lead levels in children with mental retardation of uncertain origin were not conclusive, but they delivered a warning that even modest elevations in blood lead may be associated with biochemical abnormalities in the child brain.[5] Two recent Glasgow studies have come to firmer conclusions. In one, mentally retarded children were compared with matched controls, and the lead concentration in the water from their homes and the homes of their mothers during pregnancy were measured. Lead concentrations were found to be significantly higher for the retarded group.[6] In the second study blood from new born babies used for routine testing was assayed for lead. Children with mental retardation of unknown origin showed higher blood lead levels than matched controls, domestic water being indicated as a likely source of the extra lead.[7] At least one American study has confirmed these findings.[8]

Lead has also been implicated as a causative factor in hyper-activity in children, characterised by restlessness, impatience, difficulty in concentrating, and a tendency to impulsive action. Children with hyper-activity of unknown cause showed higher blood lead levels and higher lead loss after taking a chelation compound than matched controls.[9] Moreover, such children are claimed to show an improvement in behaviour following standard lead-removing therapy.[10] The link between lead hyper-activity is confirmed by many animal experiments.[11]

Behavioural disturbances in adults have also been laid at the door of lead. A group of young adults being treated for behaviour

Figure 9.3: Comparison of Blood and Water Lead Concentrations (in $\mu mol/\iota$) in High-Water-Lead Group ($> 3.8 \ \mu mol/\iota$) and Controls

Retarded Child		Control	
Blood	Water	Blood	Water
1.98	5.6	0.71	0.1
1.44	7.7	—	0.4
2.02	8.8	1.49	0.5
1.20	5.1	0.98	2.6
—	4.4	—	1.7
1.57	6.8	—	2.1
1.82	3.9	—	2.9
—	5.8	—	1.2
1.45	4.5	—	0.6
—	5.9	1.38	1.1
1.80	5.8	1.52	0.5

Source: Adapted from M. Moore *et al., Lancet*, 2 April (1977), p.717.

disturbances and learning difficulties were found to show increased systolic blood pressure, decreased hand-eye co-ordination and shortened reaction times, all of which correlated significantly with higher lead concentration. All the lead levels measured were. however, in the normal range for US males and no subject was suspected of ever receiving undue exposure to lead.[12]

Lead has also been claimed to have a causative role in motor neurone disease[13] and multiple sclerosis,[14] although the picture in both cases is very confused. The correlation between deaths from cardio-vascular disease — stroke and heart attack — and soft water in the UK has been studied intensively, and lead may be a factor here, since soft water dissolves lead from piping more readily than hard water.[15] The case against lead is strengthened by the discovery that people in soft water areas have higher lead burdens than those in hard water districts.[16] In addition, rats given water containing lead in a concentration typical of Glasgow tap water developed biochemical and morphological changes in the heart muscle after 25 weeks.[17] The high infant mortality found in soft water areas has also been blamed on lead in the water supply,[18] as has renal insufficiency in people living in houses with lead piping.[19]

2. The Safety Factor

Kehoe found that the blood lead levels of poor Mexicans, remote from any industrial source of lead and, indeed, from any artificial source of the metal, were of the order of 0-15 μg/100 ml. These figures are not far below those for adult city dwellers in the US or UK, whose blood lead levels typically lie in the region of 10-25 μg/100 ml. Since the Mexicans' blood lead levels reflect natural contact with the metal, Kehoe suggested that they must be safe, and that urban lead levels posed no threat to human health.[20] From an entirely different scientific perspective Patterson argued that natural levels of blood lead should be as low as 0.2 μg/100 ml – about one-hundredth of present levels – suggesting that modern exposure to lead may be causing severe and widespread damage in the general population.[21] As the ensuing argument developed, it became clear that talk of 'natural' lead levels added more heat than light to the debate. The real issue is the safety margin between ordinary environmental exposure to lead and the exposure needed to produce harmful effects. Seen in this way, there is real cause for concern about present concentrations of lead, whatever we suppose 'natural' levels to be, and whatever opinion we have of the evidence mentioned earlier. Figure 9.4 (a) shows a typical distribution of blood leads in adult males in an urban environment. Indicated are Kehoe's 80 μg/100g limit, above which harm is known to occur, and the level at which lead is known to interfere with the enzyme ALA-d (δ-amino-laevulinic acid dyhydrase), which is involved in haem synthesis. This is important not because this interference is likely to lead to any harm, but because if we apply food additive standards to lead, we would have to reduce exposure so as to lower blood levels to about 4 μg/100 ml – one tenth of the lowest level known to produce any biochemical change. For comparison, Figure 9.4 (b) shows the distribution of DDT and its metabolites in the human body and the accepted threshold level. The safety margin for lead is the smallest for any substance widespread in the environment.

3. Methodology for the Measurement of the Cost-Effectiveness of Strategies

We can now see the problem more clearly. Given what we know about lead; the evidence for its sub-clinical effects and the narrowness of its safety margin, what should we do, if anything, to reduce the ordinary person's exposure to the metal? The obvious problem here is that our knowledge of the behaviour of lead is far from complete. All the evidence cited earlier may be reasonably

Figure 9.4 (a) : Typical Distribution of Blood Leads in Adult Males in an Urban Environment

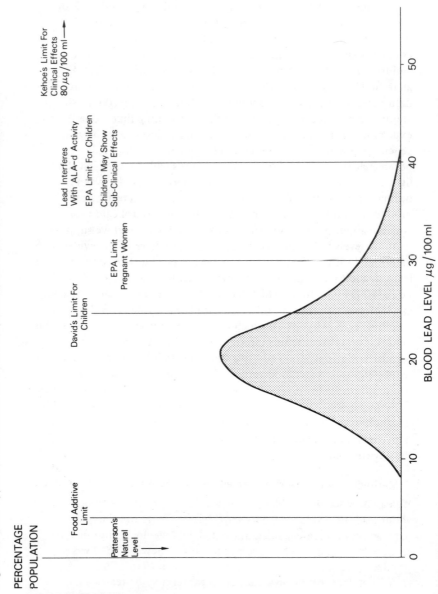

Figure 9.4 (b): Typical Distribution of DDT + DDE in Human Body Fat

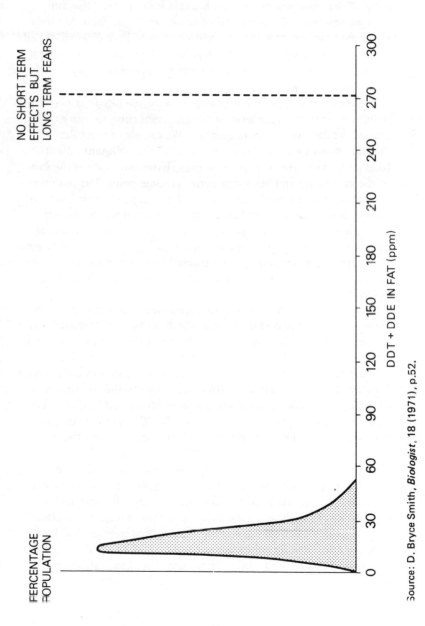

Source: D. Bryce Smith, *Biologist*, 18 (1971), p.52.

doubted and criticised. In dealing with lead we are, therefore, in the unhappily familiar position of having to make a decision in a state of gross ignorance about the relevant facts. If we decide to reduce lead levels in the environment, and such levels are in no way harmful, then we have wasted a good deal of resources. If, on the other hand, we do nothing, and lead is as dangerous as some have claimed, we add not inconsiderably to human misery. But, of course, we just do not know whether lead at concentrations found in our ordinary environment does any harm.

Figure 9.5 is a representation of how we often like to conceive of pollution control. As the level of the pollutant rises, we can expect the cost of the damage it does to increase. We can also expect that abatement costs will increase as the level of the pollutant falls. The total cost, that is the damage costs plus abatement costs, is the sum of the two curves and has a minimum at some point. The pollution level at this point is the optimum one. Lowering pollution levels to below the optimum will reduce damage costs, but not by enough to meet the extra cost of abatement. Similarly, levels higher than the optimum can be abated with a reduction in damage costs which more than offsets the extra cost of abatement. The problem of controlling the pollutant is, therefore, seen as trying to arrive at this optimum pollution level.

In the case of lead, however, this approach founders because we cannot estimate the cost of the damage done by environmental levels of the metal. The obvious approach, that of balancing the costs and benefits of controlling lead, is, therefore, ruled out. For this reason, a cost-effective approach seems required. If our aim is to lower blood lead levels in the general population, then we can find for each way of doing this its cost per unit reduction in blood lead levels (cost per 1 μg/100 ml reduction in blood lead levels). We can then compare this cost-effectiveness for each control strategy, selecting those which are highly cost-effective. It follows from what was said earlier that even for the best strategy we cannot determine whether its benefits in removing harm outweigh its cost, and this is an essential restriction of the whole cost-effectiveness approach. Nevertheless, it seems the only approach open to us. If we find a highly cost-effective way of reducing people's exposure to lead, then we may decide to bear the cost as an insurance against the kind of harmful consequences discussed earlier. If, on the other hand, all ways of lowering lead exposure have a very low cost-effectiveness, then we may decide to just live with the risks posed by environmental lead,

Figure 9.5: The Cost of Pollution

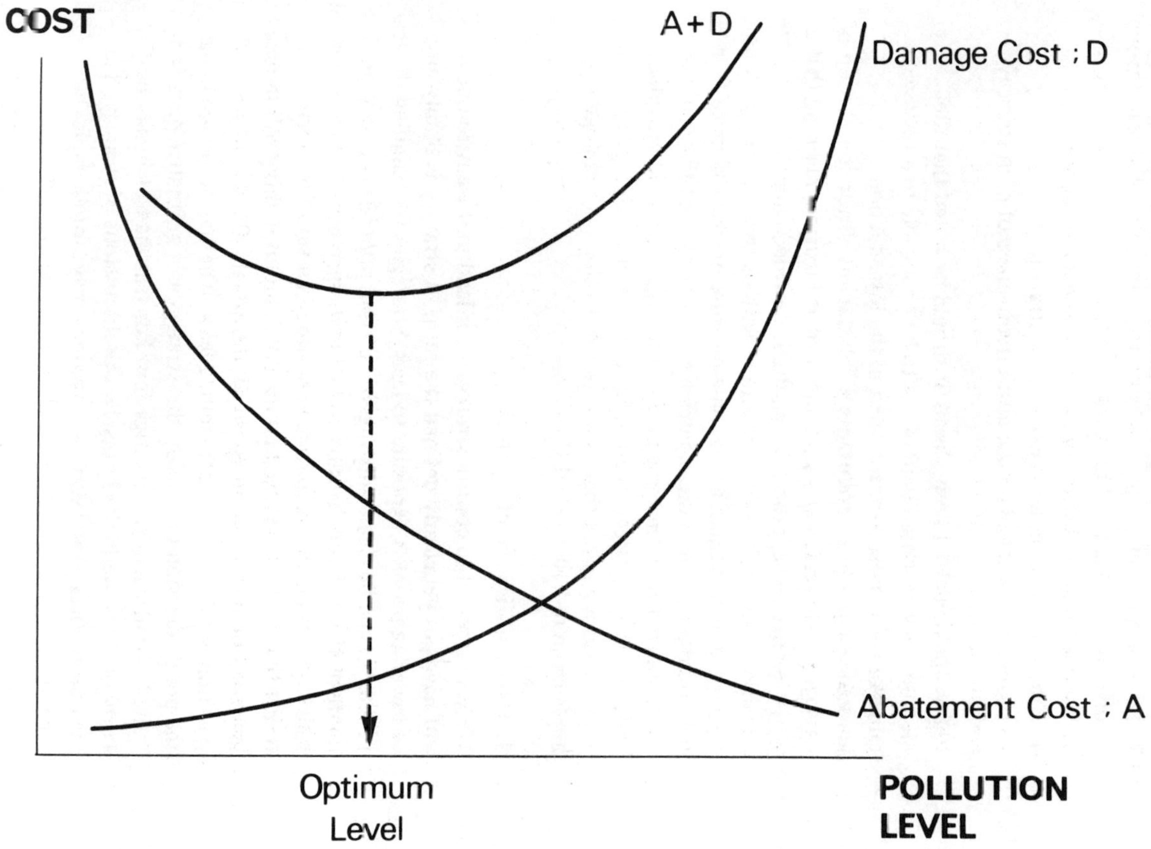

COST

Damage Cost : D

A + D

Abatement Cost : A

Optimum
Level

POLLUTION
LEVEL

the insurance premiums being too high.

We set out to measure the cost-effectiveness of control strategies for lead using a methodology of five stages.

1. Identify all possible control strategies for lead.
2. Develop a model linking exposure to various forms of lead through different channels to blood lead levels.
3. Use the model to calculate the effectiveness of each strategy.
4. Establish the minimum cost of each strategy.
5. From 3 and 4 calculate the cost-effectiveness of each strategy.

Before looking at 1 to 5 in detail, it should be noted that the methodology proposed here ought to be applicable to a very wide range of pollutants. As mentioned in the introduction, our ignorance about most pollutants precludes any direct comparison of damage costs avoided and abatement costs incurred, meaning that a cost-effectiveness approach is required. Provided enough is known to construct a model linking exposure to various forms of the pollutant through different channels to some measure of likely damage from the pollutant (such as the organism's gross burden of the pollutant or its concentration in some part of the organisms) and provided various control strategies can be costed, the methodology may be applied. Having noted that, let us return to the methodology's application to lead.

1. The Identification of Strategies

We have referred to control *strategies* for lead in the environment, but have not yet clearly defined the term. A strategy is simply any way of lowering people's exposure to lead. Strategies for handling the lead problem must be clearly distinguished from *policies*. A policy, in this context, is a political decision to tackle the problem of environmental lead by implementing a particular strategy, or set of strategies, for its control. It is a scientific fact that if doing something will reduce exposure to lead for some group of individuals, the thing in question is a strategy for controlling lead. Whether or not we make the policy decision to employ this strategy is a normative question quite beyond scientific investigation. For reasons which may be fairly obvious, we limited ourselves to discussions of strategy. This may be artificial — the very best strategy may, for example, be completely politically unacceptable, but it seems that this is an inevitable restriction on such work.

In considering possible strategies it soon became apparent that three were of particular importance; lowering lead levels in canned food, lowering the concentration of lead in water and reducing the amount of organic lead compounds added to petrol.

2. The Model

In order to assess the alleviation of the lead problem effected by each of these control strategies, a model was constructed linking exposure to lead in various forms at various body sites with an indicator of risk from the metal, such as blood lead level or total body burden of lead. Each of these indicators has its drawbacks, but blood lead is probably the most realistic. Using the model, it is possible to see what effect each strategy would have on blood lead levels (or body burden). The effectiveness of a strategy is, of course, the reduction in blood lead (or body burden) it brings about. Much more is known about the behaviour of lead in the adult male than in women or children, and for this reason our model is for healthy adult males only. This is unfortunate, since children are particularly at risk from lead and their ways of picking up the metal are very different from adults; for example, by chewing paint or sucking dusty fingers. It may, however, prove possible to apply the same methodology to children when we have learned enough about the snags from our present work.

There are two extreme types of model for this purpose, both of which we have explored. One kind merely seeks a relationship between exposure and blood lead levels (or total body burden) by an analysis of existing data. The best model of this sort has been proposed by the US Environmental Protection Agency and National Academy of Sciences. They propose a relationship of the form [22]

Blood lead = a log (total daily lead absorbed) + b

where a and b are to be found by regression from known data. Their estimate of daily lead absorption was, however, crude, and this was re-calculated.

Lead absorbed from the lung was first calculated. At least 90 per cent of such lead is from car exhaust, for which we know the approximate particle size distribution.[23] We also know the retention factors for particles in various size ranges, as shown in Figure 9.6.

Figure 9.6: Retention Factors for Particles in Various Size Ranges

Particle Size (mmd)	Distribution %	Av. Retention %
<0.1	31.7	37.5
0.1 – 0.5	63.3	30
>0.5	5.0	87.5

From this, the total retention factor for the lung was reckoned to be 35 per cent. Total lead absorbed through the lung per day, Q_L, is given by:

$$Q_L = L.B.R_L$$

where L, B and R_L are the air lead concentration, the pulmonary ventilation and the retention factor for the lung respectively.

Lead absorbed through the gut per day, Q_G, is given by:

$$Q_G = (F + W + T) R_G$$

where F, W and T are the quantity of lead in food, water and mucous transported from the lung per day, and R_G is the retention factor for the gut, taken as the widely accepted 10 per cent. The final function, therefore, has the form:

$$(Blood lead) = a \log (L.B.R_L + (F + W + T)R_G) + b$$

Given data on blood lead levels and absorption rates for a particular community, regression analysis is used to obtain the function of this form which gives the best fit. This function can then be employed to predict the changes in blood lead levels which would result from various reductions in the amount of lead absorbed. From extensive American data, the US National Academy of Sciences has suggested values for a and b of around 54.5 and 69.5 respectively.[24]

The second modelling approach attempts to provide a simulation of the flow of lead around the body, shown diagramatically in Figure 9.7. If values can be placed on all of these rates of flow we will have a pretty complete picture of the gross behaviour of the metal in the body. We have, therefore, modified the work of Lutz[25] along these lines. Lutz' model enables the total body burden of lead to be calculated for various lead inputs, along with its distribution in the blood, bone, kidney, liver and lung.

Both modelling approaches have advantages and disadvantages. The statistical approach is quick and easy, but this at the loss of insight afforded by the simulation approach. Data for the simulation approach is difficult to find in quantity and quality, but not so for the statistical approach. The simulation, is, however, more testable than the statistical model, and it has the added virtue of flexibility. We can, for example, see what happens to blood leads if kidney damage leads to a reduction in the urinary excretion rate.

Having constructed, and tested, a model of the sort described, we can calculate the effectiveness of each of the control strategies identified earlier. Figure 9.8 is a plot of lead assimilated per day *v*. blood lead level using the NAS model. The effectiveness of removing lead totally from petrol can be gauged from the figure.

If, over a particular area, this source contributes $1\mu g$ of lead per cubic metre of air, then people breathing this air assimilate on average $7 \mu g$ of lead from this source, taking average pulmonary ventilation as 20 m^3/day and a retention factor of 35 per cent. For a person with a blood lead of 30 μg/100 ml, eliminating this source of lead will lower his blood lead level to 28 μg/100 ml. The effect on blood lead will be more marked for people with a lower blood lead and, conversely, will be less for those with an original blood lead above 30 μg/100 ml.

The effectiveness of other strategies may be calculated in exactly the same way. If canned food contributes 50 μg of lead per day to an individual's diet, totally removing this source will lower his assimilated lead by 5 μg/day. For a person with an original blood lead of 30 μg/100 ml, this should effect a reduction in blood lead of about 28.5 μg/100 ml. The same argument may be used to judge the effectiveness of removing lead from domestic water supplies.

3. Cost of Strategies

(a) Lead in Food and Water

The average dietary intake of lead has been estimated to be around 140 μg per day, with between 20-40 μg/day of lead from fluid intake.[26] If lead ingestion from food is to be reduced, the most effective strategy would be to reduce lead levels in canned foods, since they contain more lead than fresh food.[27] Such a reduction could be effected in a number of ways: replacing lacquered cans by tinned ones, using tin solder instead of lead solder (as is already done for baby foods and some soft drinks), using an organic resin in place of

Figure 9.7: Lead Transport in Human Body

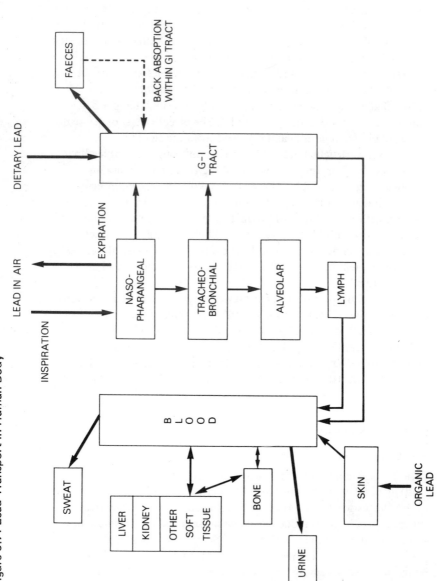

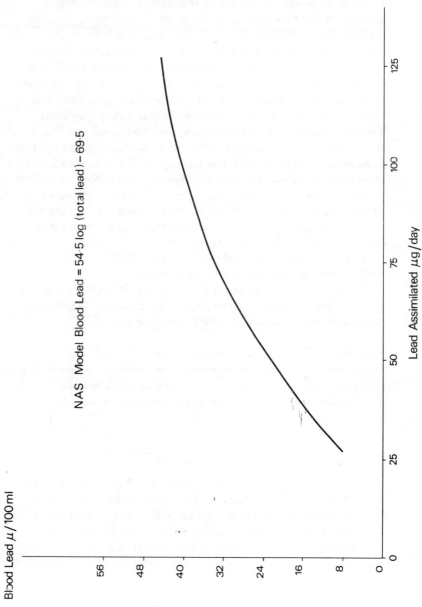

Figure 9.8: Lead Assimilated Per Day v. Blood Lead Level using the NAS Model

NAS Model Blood Lead = 54·5 log (total lead) − 69·5

the standard 3-piece can, using glass jars and so on. Accurate costing of these methods is impossible, as so many imponderables are involved such as consumer and retailer acceptance, the future cost of tin, lead, glass and aluminium, the technical feasibility of new processes, capital costs for new equipment and so on. For example, the extra cost of using tin in place of lead solder for all cans is about £8 million (1975 value) per year, but many have doubted the future availability of tin. Perhaps the most promising method would be the use of seamless 2 piece drawn and wall-ironed cans, already common as soft drink containers, in place of the traditional can. These cans have no side or bottom seam, thus eliminating leakage problems. They also weigh up to 35 per cent less than traditional cans[28] and are about 20 per cent cheaper.[29] The equipment for making these cans is, however, expensive. Metal Box have spent £11 million on four lines at their Westhoughton Plant. In addition, a higher quality tin plate is required, with problems in quality control[30] and label changes take anything up to four hours.[31] The extent to which 2-piece cans will replace conventional ones will almost certainly be determined by economic and not environmental factors.

An EEC draft directive seeks to reduce the WHO recommended limit for lead in 'first draw' domestic water from 0.3 to 0.1 mg/ℓ and in 'daytime' domestic water from 0.1 to 0.05 mg/ℓ. Figure 9.9, based on the Department of the Environment survey,[32] summarises the present state of lead in domestic water supplies.

Figure 9.9: Present State of Lead in Domestic Water Supplies

Lead in Daytime	No. of Households (million)			
Sample mg/ℓ	England	Scotland	Wales	G.B.
> 0.05	1.3	0.6	0.09	1.9
> 0.1	0.4	0.4	0.02	0.8
> 0.3	0.07	0.08	0.01	0.2

Attempts have been made to assess the contribution made by lead in fluids to blood lead.[33] It is estimated that drinking 2ℓ per day of fluid containing lead at the WHO limit of 0.1 mg/ℓ contributes 4 μg/100 ml of lead to the total blood lead concentration.

There are two ways of reducing the amount of lead in domestic supplies; the removal of lead piping and water treatment to reduce the solubility of lead. The factors which affect the solubility of lead are the pH and the hardness of the water, although the whole problem is very poorly understood at present. It appears, however, that adjustment of pH and hardness cannot be a complete answer to the problem of lead pick up.[34] Such treatment is relatively cheap and has the added advantage of being selective. Glasgow water is treated in this way, lime being added in the holding reservoir at the rate of 2-4 mg/ℓ.[35] The potential of such cheap methods for reducing lead in water is as yet unknown, although the much more expensive removal of lead piping will, of course, be completely effective.

(b) Lead in Petrol

Organic lead compounds, primarily tetra-methyl lead (TML) and tetraethyl lead (TEL), are added to petrol as anti-knock agents to prevent premature detonation of the air-fuel mixture in the cylinder. It is generally accepted that at least 90 per cent of the lead in urban air originates from the exhaust of petrol engines, and its contribution to the high levels of lead found in kerb- and road-side dust is probably of the same order. There are many ways of controlling the emissions of lead from petrol engine exhausts: reducing the amount of lead added to petrol; removing lead altogether, with associated changes in engine design to permit operation with the low octane quality fuel so produced, using a low-lead, or lead-free, fuel with an organic manganese additive to improve octane quality;[36] adding alcohol to improve fuel octane quality;[37] incorporating filters, or traps, in the exhaust system and so on. The first option, involving the alteration of refinery plant to produce the higher octane numbers required for low-lead, or lead-free, fuel manufacture will be discussed in detail to give a reasonable upper limit for the cost of reducing lead emissions from engine exhaust. However, before doing this, a brief examination of the other strategies mentioned might be of benefit.

The use of organic manganese compounds as an additive, at concentrations of 0.125 g/gallon, provides an increase of 2 Road Octane Numbers (RON). This could represent a saving of 1 per cent of the crude oil processing needed to produce high octane lead free fuel. At present it is used to tune lead free fuels to the appropriate octane quality, its economic attractiveness being greatest at low concentrations. With regard to alcohol being used as an additive, a UK Working Party stated '. . . there was no proven technical case for introducing a blend of petrol containing methanol and higher homologues as a motor spirit'. Hence, the use of alcohol in the near future seems unlikely. On the other hand, particle traps have shown promise. Tests in Europe have shown the following:

Country	Pb trapped
UK	46%
France	65%
Germany	75%

The cost of an exhaust system incorporating a lead trap is estimated to be 2 to 3 times that of a conventional exhaust system. The motor industry, however, objects to the use of traps on the grounds of increased costs and possible losses in vehicle performance.[38]

Returning now to the first strategy listed, lowering the amount of lead added to petrol, two costs are involved; the capital cost of additional refinery plant and the recurrent cost of additional crude oil. Figure 9.10 gives an estimate for the operations needed to produce leaded and lead-free petrol, the capacity of each operation being compared with the amount of atmospheric distillation required for the production of leaded petrol, which is taken as 100.

Figure 9.10: Estimated Operations Needed to Produce Leaded and Lead-Free Petrol

Process	Capacity	
	Leaded Petrol	Unleaded Petrol
Atmospheric distillation	100	103
Vacuum distillation	14.4	15.9
Catalytic cracking	10.4	10.4
Hydrocracking	0	1.11
Distillate hydrotreatment	19.4	20.0
Catalytic reforming	6.5	5.6
Catalytic reforming severe	0	4.0
Isomerisation	0	2.5
Extraction branched hydrocarbons	0	2.5
Ethylene dimerisation	0	0.5

Source: F. Porter, *Chemistry in Britain*, 10 (1974), p.61.

With regard to costs, Concawe have produced some figures for the EEC.[39] They assumed 60 x 10⁶ tons of petrol were required for 1976;

70 per cent being Premium petrol (98 RON) and 30 per cent Regular (90-92 RON). The estimated 1976 additional investment costs for all present refineries in the EEC to produce this mix of fuel, for various lead levels, are given in Figure 9.11.

Figure 9.11

Lead Content (g/ℓ)	Additional Investment ($ annual ton)
0.45	6-17
0.40	7-21
0.15	21-45

The additional production cost to manufacture 98 RON Premium and 90-92 RON Regular, in a 70-30 split, at 1976 prices is given in Figure 9.12.

Figure 9.12

Lead Content (g/ℓ)	Additional Production Cost ($ per ton)
0.45	1.7 − 8.4
0.40	2.8 − 11.2
0.15	11.2 − 22.4

However, it should be noted that rapid reductions in lead content are not feasible due to the limited size of the refining industry's reconstruction capacity. Legislation with regard to emission control should, therefore, be given with maximum advance notice and should cover as large an area as possible, e.g. the EEC. A rapid reduction in lead additives would also lead to difficulties in maintaining front-end gasoline quality[40] and the loss of the so-called lead road bonus.[41] Finally there are also environmental problems concerning the increased quantities of aromatic compounds which will be found in the exhausts produced by lead free petrols, some of which may pose carcinogenic hazards.

4. Calculation of Cost-Effectiveness

Once a minimum cost for each strategy and the effectiveness of each are known, the calculation of cost-effectiveness is elementary. In our present state of uncertainty about lead, the ranking of strategies by their cost-effectiveness inevitably involves many assumptions, but we can test whether or not these assumptions are critical to the ranking. This is best seen by considering an example. We do not know the retention factor for lead particles from petrol in the lung, but we know what limits it is likely to fall between. We can then calculate the cost-effectiveness ranking of our strategies using the upper limit and the lower limit for the retention factor. The cost-effectiveness of some of the strategies will obviously be different, but the ranking of strategies may be unchanged. If it is, then we have no need to place any priority on the discovery of the true retention factor. If, on the other hand, the ranking of the strategies is altered, then we obviously need to know the true retention factor before we can proceed to a sensible decision, and its discovery should be given priority. In this way, the methodology serves as a guide to scientific work. We can see this as a feedback loop (dotted line) in Figure 9.13.

This may well prove to be of considerable importance. Where our knowledge is as sketchy as it is about lead, it is all too easy to engage in scientific fact-finding exercises which may be altogether remote from practical affairs of policy.

This paper is a report of a study still under way and so no definite conclusions about the cost-effectiveness of control strategies for lead can be stated. We need to know more about the effectiveness of strategies, for instance we have only a hazy idea of the contribution of lead from canned food and from domestic water to total lead intake. We also need to know more about costs, for example the cost of reducing lead levels in domestic water supplies to a particular level, which varies enormously depending on whether the reduction can be achieved by water treatment or only by the removal of lead piping. When our knowledge in these areas is improved, we shall have a much clearer idea as to whether action should be taken to lower the general population's exposure to lead and about what this action should be. For the moment, we hope only to have given an idea of a methodology for the comparison of environmental control strategies and to have considered some of the difficulties involved in applying it to the particular case of lead.

Figure 9.13: Guidance of Scientific Work

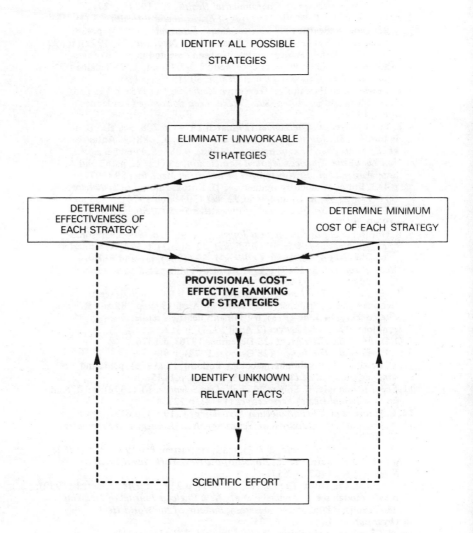

Notes

1. R. Kehoe, *Journal of the Royal Institute of Public Health*, 24 (1961)
   pp. 101, 129, 177, 203. For criticism of the threshold approach see
   H. Waldron, *Archives of Environmental Health*, 29 (1974), p.271.
2. For example, by T. Beritic, *Archives of Environmental Health*, 23 (1971),
   p.289; and A. Beattie *et al.*, *British Medical Journal*, 2 (1972), p.488;
   though see R. Kehoe, *Journal of Occupational Medicine*, 14 (1972), p.390.
   Sub-clinical peripheral neuropathy has been detected in lead workers
   whose blood lead levels never exceeded 70 µg/100 ml, A. Seppalainen
   et al., *Archives of Environmental Health*, 30 (1975), p.180.
3. For reviews see H. Waldron, *Preventive Medicine*, 4 (1975), p.135 and
   H. Waldron and D. Stofen, *Sub-Clinical Lead Poisoning* (Academic·
   Press, 1974).
4. P. Landrigan *et al.*, *The Lancet* (29 March 1974), p.708. See also B. de
   la Burdé *et al.*, *Journal of Pediatrics*, 81 (1972), p.1088; A. Antal
   et al., *Atmospheric Environment*, 2 (1968), p.383; S. Pueschel *et al.*,
   Journal of the American Medical Association, 22 (1972), p.462 and A.
   Seppalainen *et al.*, *British Journal of Industrial Medicine*, 29 (1972),
   p.443. For contradictory findings see D. Kotok, *Journal of Pediatrics*,
   80 (1972), p.57; R. Landsdowne, *Lancet* (30 March 1974), p.538 and
   J. Hebel *et al.*, *British Journal of Preventive Social Medicine*, 30
   (1976), p.170.
5. B. Gordon *et al.*, *British Medical Journal*, 2 (1967), p.480; S. Gibson
   et al., *Archives of Disease in Childhood*, 42, (1967), p.573; A. Moncrieff
   et al., *Archives of Disease in Childhood*, 39 (1964), p.1 and *British
   Medical Journal*, 3 (1967) p.174. See also J. Millar *et al.*, *The Lancet*
   (3 October 1970), p.695.
6. A Beattie *et al.*, *The Lancet* (15 March 1975), p.589; though see M.
   Heasman and D. Primrose, *The Lancet* 26 April 1975, p.982 and R. Lacey,
   The Lancet, (14 June 1975), p.1348 and Beattie's replies.
7. M. Moore *et al.*, *The Lancet* (2 April 1977), p.717.
8. O. David *et al.*, *The Lancet* (25 December 1976), p.1376.
9. O. David *et al.*, *The Lancet* (28 October 1972), p.900.
10. O. David *et al.*, Psychopharmacology Bulletin, 12 (1976), p.11, and
    American Journal of Psychiatry, 133 (1976), p.1155.
11. See, for example, E. Silbergeld *et al.*, *Life Sciences*, 13 (1973), p.1275 and
    Environmental Health Perspectives (1974), p.227.
12. L. Moore *et al.*, *Orthomolecular Psychiatry*, 4 (1975), p.61.
13. A. Campbell *et al.*, *Journal of Neurology, Neurosurgery and Psychiatry*,
    33 (1970), p.877.
14. A. Campbell *et al.*, *Brain*, (1950), p.52; H. Warren, *Practitioner*, 6 (1963),
    p.517 and H. Warren *et al.*, *Annals of the New York Academy of
    Science*, 136 (1967), p.657.
15. T. and M. Crawford, *The Lancet*, 1 (1967), p.229 and *The Lancet*, 1 (1969),
    p.699; though see T. Anderson *et al.*, *New England Journal of Medicine*,
    280 (1969), p.805, and R. Maseroni, *Bulletin of the World Health
    Organisation*, 40 (1969), p.305.
16. M. Crawford *et al.*, *British Medical Journal*, 2 (1973), p.21.
17. M. Moore *et al.*, *Scottish Medical Journal*, 19 (1974), p.155.
18. M. Crawford *et al.*, *The Lancet*, 1 (1972), p.988.
19. B. Campbell *et al.*, *British Medical Journal*, 1, (1977), p.482.
20. R. Kehoe *et al.*, *Journal of Industrial Hygiene*, 15 (1933), pp.257, 273.
21. C. Patterson, *Archives of Environmental Health*, 11 (1965), p.344, and
    12 (1966), p.137.

22. *Airborne Lead in Perspective*, Committee on Biologic Effects of Atmospheric Pollutants, National Academy of Sciences, 1972.
23. L. Danielson, *Gasoline Containing Lead*, Swedish Natural Science Research Council (1970), R. Lee *et al., Atmospheric Environmental*, 5 (1971), p.225 and Task Group on Metal Accumulation, *Environmental Physiology and Biochemistry*, 3 (1973).
24. NAS, *op. cit.*, p.66 and appendix C.
25. G. Lutz *et al., Intelligence and Project Information System for the Environmental Health Service*, 3 (1970).
26. Working Party on the Monitoring of Foodstuffs for Heavy Metals, 5th Report, *Survey of Lead in Food* (Ministry of Agriculture Fisheries and Food, 1975); R. Ainsworth *et al., Lead in Drinking Water* (Water Research Centre, Technical Report TR 43); *Lead in Drinking Water: a Survey in Great Britain* (Dept. of the Environment, Pollution Paper 12, HMSO., 1977).
27. Working Party on the Monitoring of Foodstuffs for Heavy Metals, 5th and 2nd Reports, *Survey of Lead in Food* (Ministry of Agriculture Fisheries and Food, 1975 and 1972).
28. D. Melville, Surge in US Can Making Technology, *Food Manufacture*, 51 (1976), pp.27-8.
29. An £11 million Investment in the Two Piece Tinplate Can, *Tin International*, 49 (6) (1976), pp.192-3.
30. G. Jenkins *et al.*, Demands 2 Piece Cans Place on the Properties of Tinplate, *1st International Tinplate Conference* (International Tin Research Institute Public., 530, 1977), pp.122-140.
31. R. Willson, State of the Can Making Art, *1st International Tinplate Conference* (International Tinplate Research Institute Public., 530, 1977), pp.53-68.
32. *Lead in Drinking Water: a Survey in Great Britain* (Dept. of Environment, Pollution Paper 12, HMSO, 1977).
33. P. Elwood *et al.*, Dependence of Blood Lead on Domestic Water Lead, *Lancet* (12 June 1976), p.1295; R. Ainsworth *et al., Lead in Drinking Water* (Water Research Centre Technical Report TR 43, 1977); M. Moore *et al.*, Contribution of Lead in Drinking Water to Blood Lead, *Lancet* (24 September 1977), pp.661-2.
34. R. Ainsworth *et al., Lead in Drinking Water* (Water Research Centre Technical Report TR 43, 1977).
35. M. Moore, Lead in Drinking Water in Soft Water Areas – A Health Hazard, *Science of the Total Environment*, 7 (1977), pp.109-15.
36. J. Faggan *et.al., Manganese as an Anti-Knock in Unleaded Gasoline* (Ethyl Corporation, 1975).
37. *Methane Derived Alcohols*, Report by a Working Party, Energy Paper 2 (Dept. of Energy, HMSO, 1975).
38. *Automative Emission Regulations and their Impact on Refinery Operations* (Report No. 10/77, Stichting Concawe, The Hague, 1977).
39. Ibid.
40. A. Hawkes, 'Lead in Gasoline 1 – the Issues', *Petroleum Review* (June 1971).
41. D. Hornbeck *et al., Advances of Lead in Gasoline for European Cars – the Lead Road Bonus* (SAE paper No. 750936, 1975).

10 OCCUPATIONAL CANCER AND ITS CONTROL

L.S. Levy

This paper presents an outline review of certain concepts about the nature, detection and control of cancer caused by the use of industrial chemicals and processes. Before looking at the specific area of carcinogenesis, that is, cancer caused by chemicals or physical agents, it would be useful to introduce some fundamental cancer concepts.

A cancer or neoplasm (new growth) consists of a mass of cells that has undergone changes that are fundamental, irreversible and are inheritable in that these changes are passed on from one cell generation to the next when division occurs. Essentially there are many ways and directions in which cell mutations can present themselves, but the ones we are concerned with are those in which these fundamental changes lead to a continuous and unrestrained cell proliferation.

Although in theory any cell type can give rise to a neoplasm, they tend to occur more frequently in certain tissues such as the lining of the lung, gut and cervix. As a general rule, cells which do not undergo regeneration or replacement, such as nerve cells or voluntary muscle cells, are the ones least likely to give rise to tumours. This rule may simply reflect the available number of target sites, rather than any specific susceptibility. A cell which is fully differentiated and therefore unlikely to divide cannot pass on any cancerous characteristics.

If one considers the rate of cell division occurring in the lining cells of the main airways in the lung and along the lining of the gut, it is not surprising that cancer is commonest among these organs.

The rate of growth of neoplasms varies greatly. Some may take many years to expand by any noticeable amount, whilst others may show an increase within a few weeks and extend far beyond their original point of origin. This variation in growth behaviour and rate forms the basis of a broad classification into the benign and malignant classes. Benign tumours tend to be slow growing whilst malignant tumours tend to be rapid in their growth rate. Although this classification tells us nothing about causation or site of origin, the terms are of the utmost importance in determining the severity of a neoplasm with regard to possible clinical or surgical treatment, as well as prognosis. Although there is a broad list of differences between benign and malignant tumours, probably the most important one is the ability of malignant tumours to spread to other tissues and organs not just by direct invasion, but by the formation of secondary bodies or metastases. This spread utilises the blood and lymphatic systems and typically, a small group of the primary tumour cells, having invaded the wall of a small blood vessel or lymphatic vessel, simply breaks off and becomes an embolus carried by the fluid transportation system until it reaches another organ or tissue where it becomes enmeshed and can start to expand by rapid cell division. This is why, for instance, many lung tumours produce secondary bodies in the brain, liver or kidneys.

When it comes to explaining how cancer cells arise, the best that can be said is that there is no unifying theory that can explain all the contradictions between data obtained by different investigators. To some extent, as one might expect, theories tend to reflect the interests of the investigator. Probably the most acceptable theory, or the one most easily assimilated into the field of chemical carcinogenesis, is the Somatic Mutation theory.[1] In this the transformation from normal to neoplastic cell is by damage or alteration to the nuclear DNA. This theory is conceptually satisfying, because it can explain such features as the irreversible, fundamental and inheritable nature of cancer cells. It also fits in fairly well with the idea of chemical carcinogens chemically altering the DNA by direct or indirect action to cause the prerequisite mutational events leading to a neoplastic cell. Evidence to support the Somatic Mutation theory also comes from numerous studies which have shown that many mutagens are also carcinogens and that *in vitro* many known animal carcinogens can directly interact with nuclear DNA.

A few years ago, the Zuckerman report on cancer research[2] estimated that at least 180,000 new cases of cancer occurred yearly in the UK. Estimates of mortality for the disease suggest that both in the USA and UK around 20 per cent of all deaths can be attributed to cancer. Although progress has been made in certain areas of treatment, and for certain types of cancer, overall results have been disappointing. Success has mainly been coming from treatment which leads to increases in length of survival after diagnosis, rather than a total cure.

Almost all kinds of cancer are commoner amongst older people

and the incidence rises with advancing age. However, at least half
of all cases of cancer registered in the UK arise in people who
have not yet reached retiring age. When the figures for deaths in
males of all ages in the UK were analysed a few years ago,
it was found that of those dying from cancer, the proportion that
does so during the two decades before the age of retirement
is a greater one than is the case for any other important killing
disease.

Before going on to look at the part that environmental and
occupational factors play in this cancer rate, it is important to
mention that some of this rapidly increasing incidence
of cancer seen over the last 40-50 years is in part due to the
successful treatment and cure of other potentially killing diseases.
By the very act of preventing people from dying at an early age from
infectious diseases and thereby increasing the proportion of the
population that reach middle or old age, we have created a larger target
population that is available to die from diseases of old age such as
cancer and circulatory and heart disease. This, along with better
diagnosis, must play some part in present cancer rate figures. In other
words, we have altered the pattern of death by being highly successful
in certain areas.

It is generally understood that many factors may be involved in
the development of cancer, but most importantly, many people feel
that certain extrinsic factors such as food additives, environmental
pollutants and diet are heavily implicated. These, unlike intrinsic
factors, are areas over which we have control in terms of our
exposure and for this reason need a thorough understanding if we
wish to limit their effect. Studies of cancer in regions of Africa
suggested that at least 80 per cent of cancer was environmentally
determined.[3] The International Agency for Research on Cancer
accepts as a rule of thumb that 70 to 80 per cent of cancers are
environmentally determined.[4] The evidence for such figures is
based upon differences in cancer incidence between genetically
similar populations subjected to different environmental influences.
Since factors such as genetic similarity are difficult to define and
control, it is impossible to establish whether such estimates have
any meaning. However, few people would deny that many cancers
are linked with exposure to environmental factors and it follows that a
proportion of cancers could be prevented if carcinogenic agents can
be identified and exposure to them limited or prevented.

If this logic is correct, then the role of the scientist in this area is to provide information to help decide if a material is or is not carcinogenic to man, and if it is, to then help assess at what exposure level the carcinogenic agent is going or likely to produce cancer in humans who are exposed to the material. What this really amounts to is: you can prevent a certain number of cases from occurring without necessarily understanding the mechanism by which a chemical is carcinogenic or, even less, how to go about treating it. One good reason for advocating such an empirical approach is that it is unlikely that all carcinogens operate in an identical fashion. If one compares, as an example, asbestos, a fibrous magnesium silicate which is associated with the production of both lung cancer and mesothelioma (a rare tumour of the pleural and peritoneal lining) with the highly potent bladder carcinogen, beta-napthylamine, which is an aromatic amine, it is difficult to propose any common link in the way that they can both evoke a similar neoplastic response in man.

An area of increasing concern for those in the field of Industrial Hygiene and Safety and many others is that of industrial carcinogens. Opinions differ as to the extent to which exposure to agents in the workplace contribute to the incidence of cancer. For instance, Dr John Weisberger, a vice-director for research at the Naylor Dana Institute of the American Health Foundation, speaking at a meeting last year, pointed out that factors related to an individual's life style, such as smoking and diet, could account for the largest proportion of cancers, whereas occupationally-related cancer deaths accounted for a very small number of USA cancer deaths overall.[5] In addition, according to the World Health Organisation (WHO), adequately documented cases of occupational cancer represent only a fraction of 1 per cent of the total cancer cases.[6] On the other hand, the American National Institute of Occupational Safety and Health (NIOSH) is concerned that an epidemic of industrial cancer may be beginning which is several years away from its peak.[7] In addition, it should be said that simply because documented evidence of specific cases is not available, it does not mean that they do not exist.

One of the reasons for concern over job-related cancer arises from a lack of knowledge of the long-term toxic effects of many industrial substances. Simply because we can write down the empirical or structural formula of a chemical, it does not mean that we are able to predict the effects of this material in or on the body. In many cases people are exposed to a mixture of chemicals and often transient intermediate reaction products. This makes problems of identifying risk even more difficult to resolve. According to the

WHO (1972),

> an occupational carcinogen is a carcinogen which induces cancer in men or women as a result of their occupation. Whilst some recognised occupational carcinogens are specifically identifiable physical agents, or chemical substances, others consist of variable composition. In certain instances, although it has been shown to be a proven hazard associated with a particular process, no specific compound has been identified as causative.

Science has transformed the production and development of chemicals. Naturally occuring materials can be broken down into their constituent molecules and new products synthesised whose toxicity is completely unknown, and the development of continuous flow methods and large scale processes enables such substances to be synthesised on a commercial scale. One author in 1966 estimated that 50,000 new chemicals were synthesised in laboratories in that year and that 10,000 new chemicals would become available for industrial use either in pilot or commercial quantities.[8] Another estimate in 1970 gave a lower figure of some 10,000 newly synthesised compounds in that year, only a proportion of which reached the market.[9] In this country, recent estimates give a figure of between 300-500 new materials which are produced in commercial quantities each year.[10]

It is difficult to obtain figures for the number of chemicals already in use, but it is certain to be in excess of one million. These estimates may be compared with the NIOSH estimates of the number of chemicals for which toxicity data exists. At the time their 1975 Registry of Toxic Effects of Chemical Substances was produced, NIOSH presented documentation on toxic effects for only 100,000 chemicals.[11] The data were for the most part obtained from short-term effects in animal studies. Documentation for toxic effects in humans was available for only 700 chemicals. Information on carcinogenic effects, again mostly in animals, was available for 1,545 chemicals. Clearly difficulty is arising because the study of toxicology does not seem to be keeping pace with developments in the chemical industry and furthermore, such toxicological work being done is not necessarily directed at answering the right questions about potential harm.

When it comes to the specific toxicological effect of chemical carcinogenesis the problem becomes even more complicated for a number of reasons:

1. There is no simple approach by way of looking at the chemical structure of a material and saying that it is likely to have carcinogenic properties. We cannot therefore predict from chemical structure.
2. Most carcinogens found in industry have fairly long latent periods, that is the time between first exposure and diagnosis of cancer. This can vary depending on the type of cancer produced, but as examples, lung cancers produced by certain carcinogens can take 20 years to manifest themselves in exposed workers, whilst bladder cancer caused by exposure to some of the carcinogenic aromatic amines can have a latent period of up to 40 years.
3. Continual exposure is not required, as evidenced by a group of women who were exposed to high concentrations of blue asbestos, crocidolite, during the manufacture of gas masks. They were only exposed for a period of 2 to 3 years during the early years of World War II, but cases of mesothelioma, a malignant tumour of the pleural lining did not appear until the mid 1960s.[12]

Taking these above points, it is fairly obvious that if one in error allows a carcinogen to be used in industry, it might be many years before the nature of the error is realised and even if that material is banned, there is very little one can do to prevent further cases of cancer arising in people who have already been exposed.

A fourth point is that for many industrial chemicals, Threshold Limit Values (TLV) are used as acceptable airborne concentrations in the work place.[13] These represent in general a guideline of the concentration at which the majority of people can be exposed for a working lifetime without suffering harmful effects. This implies that an appropriate graded dose-response relationship exists with a threshold below which the effect is negligible or acceptable. For carcinogens this logic does not hold true, or it has not been shown to hold true. At present we cannot talk about threshold level responses to carcinogens and therefore any level of TLV set for a carcinogen is a purely arbitrary figure. Remember, cancer unlike other toxic effects for which TLVs might be perfectly applicable, is an all or none response which is irreversible.

Before going on to look at the ways in which carcinogens are detected and controlled, the context may be set by looking at some key historical points in the story of industrial cancer.

Paracelsus in the sixteenth century, Ramazzini a little later and no doubt many others, have described diseases which we would now describe as job related cancers. However, the first full recognition and description of occupational cancer is rightly ascribed to the English surgeon, Sir Percival Pott, who in 1775 described cancrum scroti in the climbing lads of chimney sweeps. In his three and a half page chapter, Pott made two important observations — firstly he linked the scrotal cancer to an agent, namely soot and secondly he noted the time lag between first exposure, say at the age of 6 to 7 years and the onset of the disease at around the age of puberty. This as we have said is called the latent period. He also concluded that if some measure of hygiene could be observed to limit the otherwise continuous exposure to soot, then perhaps this risk could be eliminated.

In 1820, a surgeon called Paris observed skin cancer in Cornish miners and smelters of copper and tin, and he proposed arsenic as a causative agent. This observation was never confirmed, though some sixty years later arsenic was again implicated, but this time as a lung carcinogen. In the meantime, many other observations were made of skin cancer arising from occupational exposure to soot and related tar products. In addition, in the late nineteenth century, other observations were made which implicated shale oil, mineral oils and tar distillates as skin and scrotal carcinogens.

In 1879, Harting and Hesse diagnosed lung cancer in miners on the Schneeberg side of the Erzgebirge mountains in Saxony. It was later shown that a similar risk existed in the Jachymov mines on the other side of the Erzgebirge mountains. One researcher in 1944 reviewed the available data and concluded that during the years 1875 to 1939, at least 43 per cent of the miners had died of lung cancer.[14] It is now thought that the lung cancers arose from ionising radiations and this evidence is supported by the increased lung cancer rates among uranium miners of the Colorado Plateau in the USA.[15] Other forms of radiation have been implicated as cancer-causing agents, notably the ultra-violet content of sunlight and here the observed groups at risk were sailors and farmers. Up to this time, all the cancers seen had been of the skin or lung, but in 1895, Rehn recorded three workers with bladder cancer in a German dye-works. He incorrectly ascribed the risk to aniline and it was not until the 1950s that it was shown experimentally that the amine beta-napthylamine was the causative agent.[16]

In 1929 Martland reported bone cancers among World War I radium watch dial painters.[17] In 1932 Grenfell reported nasal sinus and lung cancer in Mond nickel workers.[18] In this case, both nickel carbonyl and metallic nickel and its salts were incriminated. In 1935 Lynch and Smith first reported lung cancer among asbestos workers who were already suffering from asbestosis.[19]

It is well worth noting that in all the above cases, direct causal relationships between agent and cancer were not established. Essentially, there were simply strong relationships between certain occupations or chemicals and the risk of contracting cancer. It was not until 1915 that two Japanese research workers, Yamagiwa and Ichikawa had, by continually painting the ears of rabbits with coal-tar distillate, shown that a chemical was capable of causing cancer. Not for another 18 years, in 1933, were Cook, Hewett and Hieger, starting with 2 tons of medium soft pitch, able to identify the carcinogen in coal tar as 3, 4-benzpyrene – a polycyclic hydrocarbon.[20] The above synopsis is by no means exhaustive, and in recent years other agents added to this list worthy of mention are vinyl chloride monomer (a liver carcinogen), bis (chloromethyl) ether and certain hardwood dusts.

If we are to prevent cancer in working populations by control of carcinogens, we must first identify an active agent, and having done so, then see if there is any level of that carcinogen which will not cause cancer in exposed people. If that chemical has a great economic significance, even if it is shown to be a carcinogen there may be great pressure from certain sections of the community to allow that material to be used, subject to the setting of a low Threshold Limit Value. However, there is a body of scientific opinion that states that at the present time we have no means of establishing threshold levels for carcinogens. On the other hand, it is also argued that such levels may be established which are too low to induce tumours within a human lifetime; that is, the latent period extends beyond a lifetime.

Whatever concept is used to justify a limit of exposure to a proven carcinogen, it is important to remember that so-called 'toxicologically insignificant' levels have no real validity in the field of carcinogenesis. If a carcinogen is going to be used, there is always a risk as the price of exposure.

The key question in relation to chemicals used in industry is how do we decide if a material is a carcinogen. Broadly, there are three approaches one can adopt with a view to a scientific assessment.

These are epidemiology, animal studies and short-term tests.

1. Epidemiological studies set out to examine the patterns of ill-health or mortality in populations in order to ask questions about factors which may be influential or associated in the aetiology of particular patterns or even changes in pattern. Until fairly recently, epidemiological studies have been the chief means by which the existence of a job-related cancer has been established. Such studies supply the most convincing evidence because the observations are made on people in real working situations. However, the use of such an approach as the only way of establishing a control system for potential carcinogens can be criticised on a number of counts.

The two main areas of criticism are that as a scientific method it is relatively insensitive and even more important, that it is a retrospective method of identifying carcinogens. This latter point is obviously important in that as cancers have a long latent period, until people at work develop the disease, a carcinogenic agent cannot be suspected, let alone detected by epidemiological means and further, even after exposure has ceased, people will continue to develop the disease.

On suspecting an industrial carcinogen at work, epidemiologists must carry out retrospective studies. Prospective studies may follow if required.

Essentially, retrospective studies involve researching the history of events that have been influential in causing cancer and making comparisons with other populations. In this case it will be the comparison of the incidence of either a specific kind of cancer or all cancers among the group of workers under survey with the expected incidence of cancer from figures obtained from the Registrar General's tables. There are many problems in this kind of study, such as gaps in the data required on checking back any number of years. Individual occupational histories may be severely confused by changes in modes of production and agents used or produced in the workplace. Moreover, there are factors such as movement of people between jobs in a particular workplace or workplaces as a whole.

Prospective studies do have certain advantages if it is desired to follow on from a retrospective study or even to monitor the effect of a new chemical. This is often because many of the factors which need to be taken into account have already been identified in order for the study to be set up.

One major drawback to reliance upon any epidemiological study is that this may never enable the investigator to establish a relationship. Many agents in and out of the workplace may be implicated in the causation of the common cancers such as lung cancer. Unless the agent is associated with an unusually high incidence of a rare tumour, such as angiosarcoma of the liver in vinyl chloride monomer workers, or there is a great differential between the incidence of a common cancer in people in a particular occupation and the incidence in the general population, a job related cancer may never be possible to identify.

Finally in this critique of epidemiological studies, these cannot prove a causal relationship between a chemical and a cancer. All they can do is highlight an association. This may be sufficient evidence on which to take action, but not always. In the author's specialist field of chromate carcinogenesis, epidemiology clearly demonstrated an increased risk of contracting lung cancer among people exposed to a range of chromium-containing materials in the manufacturing stages from chromite ore, but it did not tell us which of the materials was the carcinogen. In industry in general, most people are occupationally exposed to more than one chemical in their working lifetime.

2. This leads on to the role of animal studies. One can dose rats, mice, hamsters, and so on with any suspect old or new material and then compare the cancer rates of these test groups with untreated animals. In this case all factors can be controlled and the animals exposed to pure compounds, or mixtures, or whatever. However, although studies involving the use of animals have given much information relating to carcinogens, they cannot answer all questions. As a generalisation, animal studies are best used in telling us whether a material is a carcinogen – they are less useful in setting safe working levels for man. All human carcinogens, with the exception of arsenic, when tested extensively have been shown to cause cancer in experimental animals. The danger is that extensive testing might only be pursued for materials which are already strongly suspect as carcinogens. Usually, the suspicion comes from epidemiological findings.

An unknown material of no great biological activity would not necessarily be tested extensively. If one considers the case of a weak carcinogen tested in 100 rats and at the end of three years one cancer was produced, then this is a 1 per cent response, which you have just detected. If this 1 per cent response were translated into a large exposed working population, then the consequences would be horrifying. On these grounds, it must be argued that animal tests are relatively insensitive, especially if one considers that often test groups of 25 are used and thus one tumour is equivalent to a 4 per cent response. It has been argued that in order to reduce the upper limit of risk to, say, two cancers in one million in the working population, with a confidence coefficient of 0.999 would require a negative result in over three million test animals. This figure of three million is a minimum number based on the assumption that the control animals have zero incidence rate. If not, the test groups will have to be far greater.

Because it is impossible to use such large test populations of animals, high doses with smaller animal groups have to be employed to pick up carcinogenic effects. Such dose levels are often far higher than those encountered by people in the workplace. In order to try to assess the risks to man at industrial levels, and establish levels at which the risk is very low, various mathematical models have been used to extrapolate downwards from results obtained at the doses employed in animal experimentation. The problem becomes — which mathematical model fits the observations?

The Food and Drugs Administration (FDA) in the USA describes three models which fit the observations fairly well.[21] However, when extrapolated downwards, widely differing results are obtained. It was found that to reduce the risk to one in one hundred million (what was described as a virtually 'safe dose'), one model yielded a dose level of one hundredth the dose which induces tumours in one animal, whilst another model yielded a dose which is lower by a factor of 10,000. One is forced to conclude, therefore, that there is no certain way of establishing a dose which provides absolute safety and thus the choice of a method to establish a dose yielding a low level of risk is arbitrary.

Another potential problem with animal studies is that certain potential carcinogens have to metabolise in the body to produce the active carcinogen. If the test animal species chosen for an unknown compound doesn't happen to metabolise the chemical in that particular way, then a carcinogen will not be formed and thus no tumours seen.

Further difficulties associated with animal studies are that they can take many years to complete. This might delay the introduction of an important new industrial material and such tests can be extremely expensive.

3. This leads into the third category of tests known as the short-term carcinogenic testing systems.

Probably the most widely known of these is the Ames test.[22] This test is based on the assumption that many carcinogens are also mutagens. Bacterial strains are used which are treated with the test materials. Mutated colonies can be counted several days after plating out and their number can be compared to controls. Although relatively cheap and simple, there are dangers in reading too much into just one such observation. It is claimed that there is a 90 per cent correlation between animal carcinogens and positive results in this test system, but as well as the danger of false negatives, there also exists the danger of false positives. The Ames mutation system can also be used for carcinogens which need metabolic activation by the use of a liver enzyme extract.

A great deal of careful thought is required before undertaking any form of study and the safest approach usually employs a combination of studies. Epidemiology aided by animal studies is often a useful combination. The Ames mutation system and similar short-term tests will tend to find their place as pre-screening systems.

In Great Britain, Section 6 of the Health and Safety at Work Act, 1974 makes it obligatory for manufacturers and importers to ensure that materials, including chemicals, that are used at work shall be free from risk. Exactly what this means is somewhat difficult to define. In an effort to help define these responsibilities a little more clearly, the Health and Safety Executive have recently drafted a discussion document for the notification of toxic effects of substances.[23] If this is accepted, then it places on the manufacturers or importers of *new* chemicals the requirement to supply the HSE with certain toxicological information in relation to the material. This will mean that for new industrial chemicals some basic toxicological data will have to be produced. Although full carcinogenesis studies using animals are not automatically requested, some of the short-term tests of carcinogenicity are suggested as being relevant. No doubt there will be views on both sides, some perhaps saying that this might inhibit the development of new materials, whilst others might say the tests do not provide enough information to guarantee safety to those exposed. It is not expected that the number of such notifications will exceed 300 to 400 in any one year.

To summarise some of the points raised. It is at present

impossible to put a figure on the number of cancers that are caused by exposure to substances in the environment, but many feel that the proportion may be large. It is even more difficult to estimate how many cancers are due to industrial chemicals.

In industry, people are exposed to a variety of substances. There are vast numbers of industrial chemicals in use which have not been tested for their long-term toxicity and each year new products with unknown toxic effects are introduced into the working environment. It is certain that a proportion of substances in both categories are human carcinogens as yet to be identified.

Epidemiological studies are commonly used to establish a relationship between exposure to substances and human cancers. However, the use of this method can be challenged because it does not prevent human cancers and may in many cases never be able to supply the evidence to convict a human carcinogen. If such cancers are to be prevented, substances must be tested in non-human systems. These are broadly divided into two categories, those employing animals and those employing short-term submammalian models. These submammalian models are used to detect a number of different types of response to a substance, some of which may be related to carcinogenesis. These models are currently being developed and evaluated for their ability to predict whether a substance is a human carcinogen. Regardless of whether these tests are sensitive and regardless of their relatively low cost, ease of performance and rapidity with which results can be obtained, none of the tests can predict with 100 per cent accuracy which substances are or are not carcinogens.

Animal tests, with all their inherent faults, will undoubtedly continue to be used. It is felt that this form of testing is a more direct assay of human carcinogenicity since one is actually measuring tumour induction. In animal tests, it is important to produce an experimental protocol which is designed to maximise the detection of a carcinogenic response.

Once all the available evidence on the carcinogenic or mutagenic effects of any material has been gathered, it is not usually easy to predict what will happen to man. The information can be used in assessing potential harm to man, but other factors such as physical state of material, number of people exposed and the economic importance of the material may influence any decisions on whether that material is banned, or what the so-called 'acceptable' dose level is to be. One point is worth noting in this debate. If a material is a carcinogen, then it is not possible to demonstrate the existence of a working level with a zero risk to exposed human populations.

Notes

1. T.C. Bovari, *The Origin of Malignant Tumours* (Baltimore, Williams and Wilkins, 1929).
2. S. Zuckerman, *Cancer Research* (HMSO, London, 1972).
3. A.G. Oettle, 'Cancer in Africa: especially in regions South of the Sahara', *J. Nat. Canc. Inst.*, 33 (1964), pp.383-9.
4. B.A. Bridges 'Short Term Screening Tests for Carcinogens', *Nature*, 261, (1976), pp.195-200.
5. F.H. Zerkel, 'Seminar Probes Chemical and Cancer Issue, *C. and E.N.* (22 March 1976), pp.18-19.
6. L. Swaffield, 'Cutting out Cancers', *Nature*, 258 (1975), pp.94-5.
7. W. Lepkowski, 'A Headache for US Inudstry', *Nature*, 255, (1975), pp.360-1.
8. H.W. Gerarde, 'Occupational Medicine Research: Industrial Toxicology; *J. Occup. Med.*, 8 (1966), p.167, cited by Cuthbert, J.W., *Industrial Toxicology: Modern Trends – II* in Boyland, E. and Goulding, R. (eds), (Butterworth, London, 1974).
9. R.E. Eckhardt, 'Innovations in Occupational Health: Toxicological Evaluations of Industrial Chemicals', *Am. J. Public Health,* 60 (1970). p.2011.
10. Health and Safety Commission Discussion Document, *Proposed Scheme for the Notification of the Toxic Properties of Substances* (HMSO, London, 1977).
11. NIOSH, *Registry of Toxic Effects of Chemical Substances* (US Dept. of Health and Welfare, US Govt. Printing Office, Washington, DC, 1975).
12. J.S.P. Jones, S.D. Pooley and P.G. Smith, 'Factory Populations exposed to Crocidolite Asbestos – a continuing survey' in C. Rosenfeld and W. Davis (eds), *Environmental Pollution and Carcinogenic Risks* (Lyons, International Agency for Research on Cancer, IARC Scientific Publication No.13), pp.117-20.
13. Health and Safety Executive, Guidance Note E.H.15/76, *Threshold Limit Values for 1976* (HMSO, London, 1976).
14. W.C. Huper, *Recent Results in Cancer Research: Occupational and Environmental Cancer of the Respiratory Tract* (Springer-Verlag, Berlin, NY 1966), pp.125-47.
15. J.K. Wagoner, V.E. Archer, B.E. Carroll, D.A. Holaday and P.A. Lawrence, 'Cancer Mortality Patterns among US Uranium Miners and Millers, 1950 through 1962, *J. Nat. Canc. Inst.*, 32 (1964), pp.787-801.
16. G.M. Bonser, D.B. Clayson and J.W. Jull, 'The Induction of Tumours of the Subcutaneous Tissues, Liver and Intestine in the Mouse, by Certain Dyestuffs and their Intermediates, *Brit. J. Cancer*, 10 (1956), pp.653 ff.
17. H.S. Martland and R.E. Humphries, *Arch. Path.*, 7 (1929), p.406.
18. Chief Inspector of Factories, *Annual Report for 1932* (HMSO, London 1933), p.103.
19. K.M. Lynch and W.A. Smith, 'Pulmonary Asbestosis: III Carcinoma of the Lung in Asbestos Silicosis', *Am. J. Cancer,* 24 (1935), pp.56-64.

20. J.W. Cook, C.L. Hewitt and I. Hieger, 'The Isolation of a Cancer-producing Hydrocarbon from coal-tar. Parts I, II and III', *J. Chem. Soc.*, pp.395 ff.
21. US Food and Drug Administration Advisory Committee on Protocols for Safety Evaluation, Panel on Carcinogenesis, Reports on Cancer Testing in the Safety Evaluation of Food Additives and Pesticides, *Toxicol and Applied Pharmacology*, 20, (1971), pp.419-38.
22. J. McCann, E. Choi, E. Yamasaki and B.N. Ames, 'Detection of Carcinogens as Mutagens in the Salmonella/Microsome Test: Assay of Three Hundred Chemicals', PNAS, 72, (1975), pp.5135-9.
23. See note 12.

11 PROBLEMS OF DRUG PRESCRIBING IN THE NATIONAL HEALTH SERVICE

O.L. Wade

There is in this country, and in many others, increasing concern whether the extensive use of drugs in these modern times is wise, whether it is needed and whether some of the money spent on drugs might be used to better purpose. This paper is concerned with use of drugs that are prescribed by doctors in our National Health Service. Wade and Elmes showed in Northern Ireland that 95 or 96 per cent of the total cost of the pharmaceutical services was for the prescribing by family doctors and the cost of drugs used in the hospital service constituted only 4 or 5 per cent of the total drug bill. The situation is likely to be similar in England, Wales and Scotland, the hospital accounting for 10 per cent or less of the total drug bill.

Table 10.1: National Health Bill

	UK 1972 £ millions	
NHS Total cost	2732	(5.8% of GNP)
NHS Drugs	277	(10.1% of Total)

Table 10.1 shows that in 1972 the expenditure on the pharmaceutical services of the National Health Service in England, Wales and Scotland was £277 million, about 10 per cent of the total cost of the National Health Service. This proportion has remained remarkably constant since 1950, the first year for which we have data, although in recent years, with inflation, costs have increased greatly.

Table 10.2: Persons/1000 Using Drugs Over 2 Days of Survey 1963-9

NW Vermont	612
Saskatchewan	570
Liverpool	487
Buenos Aires	129
Lodz	297

Source: WHO (1972).

115

Tables 10.2 and 10.3 suggest that the use of drugs in the UK may not be as large as in some other countries, but it is difficult to compare such data because legislation, customs in drug use, the availability of over the counter medicines and drug prices vary greatly from country to country.

Table 10.3: National Drug Bill 1971

US $/Head/PA	
UK	16
Sweden	23
Germany	33
USA	37
Japan	42
France	57

Studies in Northern Ireland by Wade, Elmes and Hood have shown that the use of drugs may vary greatly, not only from doctor to doctor but from area to area. The number of units of insulin prescribed per 1,000 persons on doctors lists per month was remarkably constant, but the prescribing of oral hypoglycaemic drugs used in the treatment of elderly diabetics varied very greatly.[1] This variation was probably accounted for by differences in the emphasis placed by doctors on the use of diet: if patients keep to a strict diet they need less medication. Recent studies[2,3] of the prescribing of sleeping tablets also show great differences from area to area. Whereas the mean use was such that about 40 persons in every 1,000 on doctors lists would be receiving a nightly hypnotic, in some areas prescribing was half this level and in others, usually the more well-to-do residential areas it might be twice that level. A number of studies have been carried out comparing the use of many different types of drugs in Norway, Sweden and part of the United Kingdom. Although within each country marked differences in drug use occur, some of the differences between countries are much greater.[4,5] These and other studies arouse concern about the congruity of drug use to drug need. In some areas or some countries Vitamin B_{12},[6] hypnotics,[3] tranquillisers or hypoglycaemic drugs are little prescribed; is the higher prescribing in other areas or other countries a response to a real medical need, or is it a response to the expectation or demands of the community or to different concepts of disease and its treatment held by doctors?

Such questions are of increasing importance as the costs of health services rise and are of especial concern in countries which have State health services where the State is the dominant purchaser of drugs. In such a situation the economist finds it difficult to assess the traffic in pharmaceuticals for the normal constraints of demand and supply do not apply. Drugs for prescription are produced by industry, advertised to the medical profession, prescribed by doctors, consumed by patients and paid for mainly by the taxpayer; thus the state faces a number of parties interested in increasing the value and volume of drugs that are prescribed. The practitioner on behalf of his patient, or sometimes at the demand of his patient, prescribes medicines that he thinks are or may be efficacious, and is insulated from the cost. The patient, also insulated from cost, and naturally anxious to get the most effective treatment, is likely to imagine that the newest and most expensive drugs are the ones he needs. The manufacturers, the distributors and the pharmacists who dispense the medicines also stand to benefit financially if the value and volume of their trade increases. Price is not functioning to balance supply and demand, for high prices do not lead to a reduction in monetary returns. Such circumstances give rise to a reasonable concern that it might be possible for a health service to institute economies in its use of drugs without impairing the standard of health care given to patients. In the light of this concern it is instructive to look at some of the measures which have been or might be used to encourage economy in prescribing in our National Health Service.

1. Influencing the Prescriber

It is claimed that if medical students were taught more about the cost of drugs and the need for economy and if measures were sought to acquaint general practitioners and hospital consultants in a simple and striking form with the efficacy and relative costs of drugs, the prescribing costs of the NHS would be substantially reduced. Those who have had experience of undergraduate and graduate teaching, however, would not expect such efforts to be more than marginally effective. In education it is not what is taught that is important, it is what is learnt. Experience has shown that students and doctors will learn readily enough about what they think is important to them, about drugs, the use of drugs, the mechanism of action of drugs or adverse reactions to drugs, but they cannot be expected to take a major interest in drug costs from which they are insulated. The

Department of Health and Social Security (DHSS) has for many
years bombarded doctors with information about the cost of drugs,
advised on equivalents or near equivalents to proprietary
medicines, urged the use of non-proprietary rather than proprietary
medicines, encouraged the use of generic names instead of the more
easily remembered trade names and arranged lectures to stiffen
the resistance of doctors to the claims of advertisements and the
persuasion of salesmen: but all to little effect.Indeed it would be
interesting to discover whether DHSS can justify the costs of its
campaigns by showing that they have led to substantial savings. The
information about drug costs that they circulate seems unlikely
to make much impact on doctors who are being simultaneously
subjected to the deluge of advertisements from drug companies
which pour through their letterboxes, and the visits of
persuasive salesmen.

There is no doubt, however, that if a compact standard
reference book like the British National Formulary gave clear
information of the cost of generic preparations and the cost of
proprietary preparations many doctors would prescribe the generic
preparations: they are often considerably cheaper by a factor as much
as five than the proprietary preparations and in many instances
would be entirely adequate.

2. Disciplining the Prescriber

Since 1950 the Pricing Bureau has at regular intervals analysed the
prescribing costs of every doctor who is informed of his costs in
relation to the average of doctors in his area. Those whose
prescribing costs are unduly high, usually more than twice the
average of other doctors in the area, are visited by Regional
Medical Officers. After such a visit doctors usually reduce the cost
of their prescribing but if they persist they may be called to appear
before a Local Medical Committee to justify their prescribing. The
Local Medical Committee may advise that monies be withheld from
a doctor's remuneration. This is a clumsy machinery and is seldom used
except where there has been a gross or stupid abuse. The costs of
carrying out the analyses and of visiting the doctors may not be
justified by any reduction in the prescribing costs that result, for
the system causes resentment and ill feeling among some doctors
and may be counter productive in terms of their willingness
to co-operate with the DHSS. There is a story, probably apocryphal
about one doctor who was visited by a Regional Medical Officer.

He subsequently wrote to the 3 per cent of patients on his lists
for whom his prescribing had been most expensive requesting
them to transfer to other practices. He not only cut down his
prescribing costs dramatically but he reduced his work load by
25 per cent.

3. Prescription Charges

In 1952 a prescription charge was imposed. Initially it was 1s per
prescription form but in 1953 it was increased to a 1s per item.
The imposition of prescription charges was initially opposed
vigorously by the British Medical Association, but when in 1963
there was a proposal that they should be abolished there was a
volte-face: anxiety that nothing should interfere with the supply of
drugs that a patient needed had been replaced by anxiety that
withdrawal of the charges would increase the number of
unnecessary visits made to doctors for minor needs.

In Northern Ireland neither the imposition, the removal of
prescription charges, their reimposition nor changes in the charges,
seemed to make much difference to the rate of increase in the costs
of prescribing over a period of 20 years. Indeed on reflection a
fixed prescription charge dependent on the number of items
prescribed would not be expected to have very much effect
on the major cause of the increased drug bill which is the increased
cost of each item. If the prescription charges were varied according
to the cost of the drug, they might make some impact on the cost of
prescribing but it would very fairly invite accusation of charging the
sick and would be politically unacceptable.

4. Regulation of Drug Prices

In 1957 the Ministry of Health entered into an agreement with the
Association of the British Pharmaceutical Industry for a scheme of
price regulation. The main features of the scheme were

1. If a preparation had substantial exports the home price should be
   no more than the export price.
2. If a preparation, not substantially exported, had an exact standard
   equivalent its price should be no higher than the equivalent.
3. For other preparations the maximum price should be calculated by
   a specially constructed trade price formula.

New preparations were excluded from this scheme for four years if they

were the results of research and for two if they were not. By 1959
prices had been agreed for some 88 per cent by value of all
preparations falling within the scope of the scheme.

This scheme with modifications has continued since. It is
difficult to assess its efficacy but it would appear to have been
very successful if the prices of drugs in Britain are compared with
prices in other countries. It works because both parties concerned
wish the scheme to work. The state cannot demand prices so low
that it exposes itself to the accusation that it has driven drugs off
the market or has made the discovery of new drugs more difficult:
the pharmaceutical industry cannot be indifferent to allegations that
it is profiteering at the expense of the sick.

5. Restrictions on Advertising

Many believe that the excessive and insistent claims made in drug
advertisements encourage unnecessary prescribing. In Britain the
Medicines Commission now insists that there is a data sheet published
for every drug by the firm that markets it. The data sheet has to be
agreed by the Licensing Authority in consultation if necessary with
the Committee on Safety of Medicines. It is illegal for a firm to
promote a drug for any purpose other than those set out in the
data sheet.

It is however difficult for both the Licensing Authority and
the Association of the British Pharmaceutical Industry which has
a strict code of advertising to maintain a surveillance of advertisements
and it is almost impossible for them to control what the firms'
representatives say to doctors. Some hospitals insist that representatives
are only allowed to call on members of the hospital staff, especially the
junior medical staff, if they have made an appointment. Some
hospitals restrict the generous 'hospitality' which firms extend to
the residents' mess. Others although disliking this 'hospitality'
believe, as indeed do some of the best firms, that the good sense
and competence of young graduates leads them to discredit firms
that use such methods.

There has also been concern that many reputable medical
journals now depend to an excessive amount on their advertising
revenue and accept advertisements which are unworthy of their
status. This may be true but an editor is understandably likely to be
influenced not only by financial considerations but also by a

profound dislike of any censorship or interference with freedom of speech. More disturbing is the recent rash of medical newspapers and magazines sent unsolicited and for no payment to doctors, which are media both for advertisements and for articles which encourage the use of drugs.

In recent years firms have made a practice of supporting post-graduate meetings and symposia. It is difficult to draw a line between what is reasonable and what is excessive. There is no doubt that many doctors would not come to post-graduate meetings so readily were it not for the meals and hospitality that are supplied and post-graduate education has benefited from this policy.

Sometimes however the hospitality is excessive: free transport to a desirable resort, perhaps abroad, for both the participants and their wives, predominance of papers that are favourable to the products of the firm concerned and gifts that are inappropriately generous are not unknown

What is most wanted is that the restrained and reasonable behaviour of the best firms should be accepted by all. This is probably best achieved by persuasion rather than legislation, and would probably be best achieved if doctors evinced more concern about the standards of advertising and refused to be influenced by excessive promotion.

6. Nationalisation of the Pharmaceutical Industry

Nationalisation of the pharmaceutical industry or of part of the industry has been suggested. This suggestion may have a political mileage but it is hard to see that it would bring the price of drugs down substantially. The profit obtained on drugs must usually represent only a fraction of the final prices. The high standards of purity, the rigorous testing, the demands of the code of good manufacturing insisted on by the Licensing Authority and the nature of research and development, mean amongst other things that this industry employs a higher proportion of university graduates and skilled technicians than any other major industry in the UK. Whether a company is privately owned or is nationalised, producing high quality modern drugs is expensive.

7. Restrictions on Prescribing

Numerous proposals for restriction of the drugs or preparations that may be prescribed by doctors have been made. The most recent were outlined in a Bill, Medical Practitioners (Restriction of Right to Prescribe) put before Parliament in May 1976 which would restrict doctors to simple and innocuous remedies unless they could show that they were regularly attending post-graduate instruction on drugs.

In New Zealand, Australia and Denmark tariff systems have been introduced. Drugs are classified into categories such as 'lifesaving', 'important' and 'others' (Denmark) for which patients pay respectively nothing, a small charge or a large charge. There appear to be no major complaints of inadequate medical treatment from either the public or doctors in countries which have a tariff scheme, but such systems are expensive to administer. There is some argument about the savings achieved but these are probably substantial.

Wade and McDevitt[7] examined the use of the British National Formulary (BNF) by prescribers in Northern Ireland. They found that only about 12 to 21 per cent of prescriptions were for preparations in the BNF, but that more than 91 per cent of prescriptions could have been written from it, with, in their opinion, no loss to the patient. At the prices of that time this would have saved the Northern Ireland Health Service £1 million in a total drug bill of £4.1 million. If such a policy were to be imposed on the whole UK, although it would mean that many fewer preparations of drugs were prescribed than at present, it would seem likely that the prices of those that were prescribed would rise. Although there may be good therapeutic reasons for persuading doctors to prescribe from the BNF it would be wrong to assume it would reduce the drug bill radically.

In their survey Wade and McDevitt compared the prescribing of some 'high cost' doctors with 'low cost' doctors. The difference in costs were only marginally due to any difference in the drugs or preparations they prescribed and neither used the BNF very greatly. The different cost was mainly due to the large quantities that the high cost doctor prescribed on each prescription compared with the smaller quantities, usually enough for only a week or ten days which were prescribed by the low cost doctor. If the high cost doctors thought, and some of them appeared to, that by prescribing large amounts they increased the period of time before the patient visited their surgery again it would appear that they were mistaken. In practices of the same size the number of visits from patients for prescriptions were as frequent each month as in the low cost practice. In 1954 the New Zealand Health Authority introduced a restriction on the maximum quantity that could be ordered by a doctor at once, and limited this to the amount necessary for fifteen days treatment with the possibility of one repeat. However the conditions of service of doctors are different in the UK from New Zealand and although doctors should be strongly encouraged to restrict the quantities they prescribe, it would not be easy to supervise a mandatory system and special arrangements would have to be made for a large number of patients with long term diseases such as diabetes, hypothyroidism, epilepsy or asthma.

A cogent reason for doctors to restrict the quantities they prescribe is the evidence of surveys which show what a large proportion of prescribed medicines are not used by patients. They are kept in the house sometimes to be used inappropriately for another illness or by another member of the household and sometimes, for they are seldom left locked in a medicine cupboard, to cause accidental poisoning to a toddler or to be used in self-poisoning by someone in distress or misery. Dunnell and Cartwright[8] in a survey of 1401 persons found that 45 per cent of the prescribed medicines in the home had not been used at all in the month before the interview and 25 per cent had not been used in the previous six months. Thirty-five per cent of the containers of medicines that had not been used during the previous year were three quarters full.

A particularly worrying feature of general practice in recent years has been the increasing habit of many doctors to sign repeat prescription forms which have been filled in by a receptionist without the doctor seeing that patient at all. For a few patients well known to a practice who have a regular need for medicines this may be acceptable. That so many patients now receive repeat prescriptions without question for months or even years without seeing their doctor, is not only bad medical practice but is also the cause of a waste of money, for many of these prescriptions are unnecessary.

8. Financial Incentives to Economise

Ways of providing doctors with a financial incentive to prescribe economically have not been used since the NHS was established in 1948. But when the National Health Insurance scheme was inaugurated in 1912 arrangements were made so that 2s out of the 9s capitation fee were set aside to form a drug fund. If in any area the cost of drugs fell below 2s per head the difference up to a maximum of 6d was added to the remuneration of the doctors in the area. If the cost exceeded 2s per head the pharmacists accounts were scaled down.

This 'floating sixpence' was abolished in 1920. The scheme must have been difficult to administer, and but for the fact that only a limited section of the employed persons in the population were covered by the insurance scheme, it would surely have eventually generated ill feeling between pharmacists and doctors and between the doctors in an area.

After Wade and McDevitt[7] had completed the survey in Northern Ireland which showed that a saving in pharmaceutical costs might be achieved if doctors prescribed more from the British National Formulary, it was suggested that a sum of £75 a quarter might be paid to all practitioners who could show that 75 per cent of their prescriptions were from the BNF. It is a pity that this suggestion was not accepted for a trial period. It would have shown whether an incentive of this type did or did not achieve what was its main aim; to persuade doctors to think continually of economy in the prescribing of drugs.

9. Prescribing Budgets

The idea that doctors should have a drug budget has to date only been considered, and usually rather perfunctorily, in hospitals. With the present restriction of funds in the hospital service it has become increasingly clear that new developments can only take place at the cost of reducing existing commitments and there is now beginning to be discussion, argument and decision about economies. In some hospitals the medical and pharmacy staffs are beginning to examine the use of drugs in their hospital in order to reduce the drug bill. If there is a ward pharmacy service it is suggested that pharmacists who are far more knowledgeable than doctors about drug costs, should be requested to keep the medical staff, and particularly the junior medical staff, alerted to the cost of the drugs they prescribe, and especially about the cost of expensive drugs such as antibiotics, corticosteroids and cytotoxic drugs.

The need for the hospital pharmacy to supply drugs to outpatients has also been questioned. This may occasionally be of real importance to patients but it is often no more than a convenience for them. Although its restriction might help a hospital budget and allow a reduction of pharmacy staff, the Health Service would eventually have to meet the cost of the drugs after they had been prescribed for the patient by his own doctor. The cost of prescribing outside hospital is greater than the cost in a hospital where the pharmacy is often able to purchase at a discount and has none of the overheads of the pharmacy shop in the High Street.[9]

There has to date never been any discussion in the Health Service of the possibility of establishing a prescribing budget for general practitioners. Yet this would seem on reflection to be a measure that might effectively reduce the drug bill of the NHS. Each doctor might be given a 'drug allowance' of £100 or £500 per 100 persons on his list to meet the costs of his prescribing. If he prescribed in excess of this, other than in exceptional circumstances, the excess would be met from his practice: if he prescribed within his budget the savings would accrue to his practice to be available for other services. In a scheme of this sort there would then be a strong incentive for:

1. The doctor to know the cost of every item he prescribed
2. The doctor to question the need for every prescription he wrote
3. The drug industry to be intensely competitive in its drug prices
4. The drug industry to concentrate its research and development on those products which would be likely to be a real therapeutic advance.

This suggestion is not as revolutionary as it first appears. The principle is already established in a slightly different context where the practitioner is reimbursed for most of his practice expenses with a sum calculated by averaging the costs of a sample of practices. These average costs are obtained by examining the claims submitted from a sample of practices to the Inland Revenue. Practices which keep their costs below this average will gain a profit whereas those where the costs are greater than the average have a loss.

Conclusion

Modern drugs have brought great benefits to mankind: doctors would not like to practice medicine without penicillin, cortisone or modern vaccines. These benefits would not be available but for the endeavours and skills of the pharmaceutical industry because the production of drugs demands great expertise and rigorous standards of production.[10]

There is no doubt however that substantial economy in the prescribing of drugs could be achieved: it would not harm patients and it would benefit other sections of the Health Service which are short of money. What is needed is a change in attitude.

There has been since the beginning of the National Health Service a firm and reasonable conviction amongst doctors that the treatment a patient gets should be a matter of decision by a doctor. In their desire to defend this reasonable tenet doctors have resented any criticism of their prescribing, including any criticism of the costs that they incur.

In these times of financial stringency for our country, there is likely to be a reduction in the monies available for the Health Service. It would seem wise for doctors to accept this unpleasant fact and agree to arrangements that reduce the costs of drug prescribing but leave them professional freedom. Unless they do this themselves restrictions may be imposed upon them by persons who do not understand how important professional freedom is to the health of medicine.

Notes

1. O.L. Wade, 'The computer and drug prescribing' in G. McLachlan and R.A. Shegog (eds.), *Computer in the Service of Medicine* (Oxford University Press, London, 1968).
2. P.C. Elmes, H. Hood and O.L. Wade, 'Prescribing in Northern Ireland. Methods of analysis', *Ulster Medical Journal*, 45 (1976), p.56.
3. P.C. Elmes, H. Hood, C. McMeekin and O.L. Wade, 'Prescribing in Northern Ireland. Study No.1. Sleeping tablets', *Ulster Medical Journal*, 45 (1976), p.166.
4. U. Bergman, P. Elmes, M. Halse, T. Halvorsen, H. Hood, P.K.M. Lunde, F. Sjoquist, O.L. Wade and B. Westerholm, 'The measurement of drug consumption. Drugs for diabetes in Northern Ireland, Norway and Sweden', *European Journal of Clinical Pharmacology*, 8 (1975), p.83.
5. A. Engels and P. Siderius, 'The consumption of drugs. Report of a study 1966-7', Unpublished WHO Working Document, EURO 3101 (Copenhagen, 1968).
6. A.L. Cochrane and F. Moore, 'Expected and observed values for the prescription of vitamin B12 in England and Wales', *British Journal of Preventive and Social Medicine*, 25 (1971), p.147.
7. O.L. Wade and G.D. McDevitt, 'Prescribing and the British National Formulary', *British Medical Journal*, 2 (1966), p.635.
8. K. Dunnell and A. Cartwright *Medicine Takers, Prescribers and Hoarders* (Routledge & Kegan Paul, London, 1972).
9. L.J. Opit and R.D.T. Farmer 'Cost of dispensing in the pharmaceutical services' *Lancet*, i (1974), p.160.
10. Department of Health and Social Security, *Guide to Good Manufacturing Practice* (HMSO, London, 1976).

12 THE RATIONAL PRESCRIBING OF MEDICINES

Peter A. Parish

Before the rational use of medicines available upon prescription is discussed, it is essential that the prescribing and use of medicines be put into a social context. These are very complex social activities in which numerous social, economic and psychological factors affect a doctor's decision to prescribe a particular medicine to a particular patient, and affect the patient's decision about whether, when, and how to take a prescribed medicine. What must be recognised is that the doctor has freedom to prescribe what he thinks is appropriate for his patient: a freedom often referred to as 'Clinical Freedom', which is jealously guarded by doctors and means that under the protective umbrella of the medical profession a doctor is able to be an idiosyncratic prescriber.

The freedom or autonomy of the patient must also be recognised; the degree of which is evident from studies which have demonstrated that many patients do not adhere to instructions given to them about the use of a prescribed medicine. Furthermore, the collection of unused medicines from households indicate that huge quantities of medicines are prescribed far in excess of what the patients themselves thought was appropriate. Such studies demonstrate much wastage and yet demand by patients is often blamed for the increasing volume of medicines prescribed by doctors. But in talking about demand from patients it must be realised that expectations are usually determined by the actions of doctors. For example, if doctors label symptoms produced by everyday problems of living as medical problems requiring a medicine, they define for their patients a way of coping with the stresses and strains of their everyday way of life. Doctors ought not then to complain about the 'demand' by patients for medicines. But of course doctors have their own expectations: they too have been led, by the marketing activities of manufacturers and suppliers of medicines, to recognise and label patients' problems as medical ones requiring medicinal treatments. Clearly doctors' actions contribute to the frequency of issue of prescriptions and the volume of medicines prescribed, which subsequently lead to wastage.

The British Department of Health & Social Security, as keeper of the public purse, attempts to exercise economic control over such activities. This is a difficult task when it is realised that the budget for the supply and dispensing of medicines is open ended and that the Department has to deal with profit making manufacturers, suppliers and dispensers of medicines whilst relying upon entrepreneurial general practitioners to act as gate-keepers to the free services and facilities provided by the National Health Service.

General practitioners in their role as gate-keepers have to make many and varied decisions about treatment, and in a few minutes per patient can open inflationary flood-gates which create demands upon the system out of all proportion to the health needs of the community they serve. The cost of medicines is part of this flood and we must question whether such expenditure is warranted, not only in monetary terms but also in terms of overall ratio of benefits to risks for those receiving treatment.

Against such a background it is evident that the problems we face in the prescription and use of medicines have not been created by any one group and are not going to be solved by any one group. They are, as has been indicated above, social acts which reflect the consumer 'throw-away' society in which we live. But, clearly, generous prescribing leads to unnecessary costs and it is therefore important to recognise that economic prescribing is dependent upon the adherence of the doctor to accepted standards of prescribing practice. If the doctor is responsible in the way that he prescribes medicines and attempts to seek their appropriate and safe use then his prescribing should inevitably be more rational.

Some of these standards may be defined further. To be a *responsible* prescriber the doctor should be responsible for his prescribing actions to his peers and more importantly to his patients. This means we ought to consider moving towards local multi-disciplinary peer group reviews of medicinal treatments and develop a system of informed consent from patients. This will require education of doctors and patients about the expected benefits and risks of a particular regimen.

To be a responsible prescriber the doctor should also have adequate knowledge about the patient he is treating, the patient's disorder, and the medicines he prescribes. He should also keep adequate records, and provide adequate instructions to the dispensing pharmacist. He should inform the patient of the reasons why he is prescribing a medicine, give an indication of expected benefits and risks, and provide the patient with adequate instructions on how and when to take the prescribed medicine or alternatively make arrangements for the dispensing pharmacist to provide such information.

To be *rational*, prescribing should be sensible and not extravagant and any medicinal treatment should be based upon what may be tested by accepted canons of scientific enquiry, allowing for the various factors which may influence the outcome of treatment. I suggest that four criteria should be applied to prescribing; these are that doctors should attempt to make medicinal treatments more *Effective, Appropriate, Safe* and *Economic*. These are inter-dependent criteria and each criterion should not be considered in isolation.

An *effective* medicine is one which has been demonstrated to produce more benefits than risks for whatever reason it is used. However, in the natural progression of any disorder, there are many factors other than the taking of a medicine which determine response to treatment. The prescribing doctor should not too readily associate with treatment any improvement in the patient's condition without prior knowledge of the natural history of the disorder without medical intervention, and without obtaining information back from the patient as to whether he improved and as to whether he took the prescribed medicine as directed.

Appropriate treatment is what will benefit a particular individual with a particular disorder at a particular time under particular circumstances. By this I imply that a doctor should consider that a patient, his symptoms and his environment are in a state of constant change. Any of these may change over time and influence the appropriateness of treatment. The specific medicine used should also be appropriate for the patient and the disorder being treated. It must be given in an appropriate form and dosage, by the most appropriate route, at the most appropriate intervals of time and for the most appropriate duration of time. This requires the application of special knowledge about the probable actions and formulations of a particular medicine in the treatment of a particular patient.

There is no such thing as a one hundred per cent *safe* medicine, every treatment is a balance between benefits and risks for the individual being treated. This means that in addition to a prescribed medicine having had to meet the safety requirements of the statutory authorities, its safety must also be considered when using it in a particular individual with a particular disorder. There are risks to the use of any medicine and these risks increase if it is used inappropriately. Many adverse reactions to medicines could have been predicted and prevented and here it must be emphasised that one deficiency in the drug related health service is the gap between knowledge which is available about medicines and the application of this knowledge to the treatment of patients. Another deficiency is in our knowledge about the extent of adverse reactions to medicines. Yet such information should be available if we are to make more appropriate and safe the use of medicines. Furthermore, the use of many medicines is based more upon anecdote, clever marketing and fashion than upon scientific evidence of effectiveness.

However, the provision of information alone will have little influence unless the prescribing doctor assimilates it and uses it as knowledge when making decisions about medicinal treatments. Clearly we need to improve education and communication and relationships if these gaps are to be closed.

Prescribing should be *economic* if it is appropriate, effective and safe. By the use of expensive promotional gimmicks, 'me-too' drugs, expensive combination products, the association of novelty with effectiveness, and by large volume and frequent prescribing, the doctor will increase the cost of his prescriptions but will not ensure that treatment is any more appropriate or safe.

There are few who doubt that the prescribing of medicines could be very much more rational. As has been indicated, there is need for education, not only of doctors but of other health professionals and patients. Methods of communication must be improved so that information and knowledge that is generated by the drug companies and researchers is disseminated effectively and applied to treatment decisions. It has also been suggested above that the problems we face are not going to be solved by any one group. Some of these problems are that: the dissemination of information by drug companies is confusingly tied up with sales promotion, every prescription representing a sale. Continuing education of doctors about medicines is principally in the hands of drug companies. The Department of Health & Social Security, because of respect for the clinical freedom of doctors has ignored inappropriateness and lack of safety in prescribing. Because their education is principally concerned with diagnosis, doctors are almost demotivated from learning about medicines. They appear not to recognise that it is by advances in medicinal treatments that most of their practice of medicine will develop. Nurses receive minimum education about medicines, pharmacists whilst having their education expanded have had their role in the Health Service reduced to the often simple task of dispensing already compounded and packaged medicines. The consumer has been left almost in total ignorance of the medicines he/she takes.

Recommendations To Make Prescribing More Rational

Prescribing could be made more rational if some of these problems are tackled using a multi-disciplinary approach from doctors, pharmacists, epidemiologists and educationalists. In our main teaching hospitals centres for education, research and service in the use of medicines should be developed. The core staff of these centres should be specially trained physicians (clinical pharmacologists) and specially trained pharmacists (clinical pharmacists.) Their main function would be: to develop effective relationships and communications in order to provide education about medicines to doctors, pharmacists, nurses, other health care professionals and consumers in their region; to carry out research on the actions, effects and uses of medicines; to monitor for adverse reactions to medicines, and to provide a medicines information and medicinal treatment advisory service.

13 PUBLIC POLICY AND INNOVATION IN THE DRUG INDUSTRY*

H.F. Steward

The influence of public policy on the research and innovation process in science-based industries has emerged as an important area of concern and controversy. The growth of legislation on hazard control, environmental standards and consumer protection is one of the factors prompting this. The increased government intervention in these spheres is itself a reflection of the failure of the market mechanism to ensure harmony between technological change and social needs. The drug industry has emerged as a focus for the discussion over public policy and innovation because of its research intensity and the fact that as an industry it is subject to quite a developed structure of control through the Prices Regulation Scheme and the Medicines Act. A recent conference of industrial managers was held on precisely this theme[1] and the *Financial Times* recently commented that the most crucial issue currently facing the pharmaceutical industry was how to maintain 'thorough and effective research and development programmes in spite of increasingly stringent government controls over drug safety, efficacy and . . . prices'.[2]

Before examining the pharmaceutical industry let us look at the schematic description of the operation of decision-making on technological change given by Baram[3] (Figure 13.1). Although this raises many interesting points about the interaction of influences on decision-making, the main point that needs to be stressed is that control, whether private or public, can be exerted at two distinct points in the innovation process; either over the inputs to or the outputs from research and development programmes. The influence of public policy at either of these points may be general or specific. For example, the allocation of resources to R & D in general can be encouraged by favourable price and patent policies. The allocation of resources to specific, desired research programmes, however, could only be achieved by a more direct form of public intervention. Likewise general control over the output of innovation could be exerted by increasing the knowledge of consumers so that the market operates more effectively (for example

Figure 13.1: The Operation of Decision-making on Technological Change

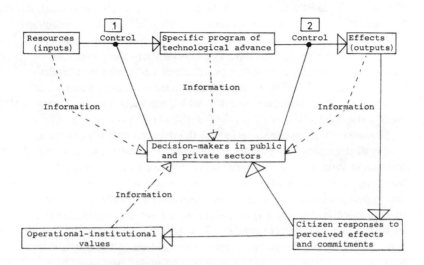

by controlling advertising and providing independent information). Specific control can be implemented through, for example, the legal requirement for every new product to be licensed on the basis of safety and efficacy.

As well as this distinction between the general and specific influences of public policy it is important to stress a further characteristic. This is, that although the direct effects of particular policies are exerted at the two distinct points identified, significant indirect effects may also manifest themselves. Control over the choice and scale of research (resource allocation) will obviously affect the new drugs discovered and introduced (innovative output). Conversely, control over the introduction of new drugs may well, over a longer term, have some influence over the choice of research projects. The main problem with such indirect effects is that they are extremely difficult to predict and some of their unexpected consequences may contradict the goals of the original policy.

Two examples of precisely this problem have been suggested. Government policy on drug pricing may serve to encourage industrial research in general, yet it fails to specify which projects are desirable. Industrial firms in the words of Mr J. Spink still remain 'fairly free agents in the way in which we conduct our search for new therapeutic agents'.[4] The indirect consequence of a policy aimed at producing conditions favourable to the development of important new medicines may in fact encourage research which is commercially attractive but socially unnecessary such as that resulting in drugs similar to those already available. The Labour Party's working group on the industry argued this point when it observed that 'under the Voluntary Price Regulation Scheme it is impossible to be sure that all research and development activity, which can be charged as a cost, is socially useful'.[5]

The second example is the effect of the requirements for pre-market testing of the safety and efficacy of new drugs in pushing up the cost of research in general. A policy designed to improve the effectiveness of new drugs may as a result have the indirect effect of further discouraging industrial innovation in economically unattractive, but socially important areas. The NEDO Report 'Focus on Pharmaceuticals' suggested that 'certain rare conditions occurring in the developed countries and some diseases of common occurrence in the less developed countries' were such a case and estimated that in 1970 a return of £20 million was the minimum justifying a new product introduction.[6]

Consideration of the influence of public policy on drug innovation points to the basic characteristics of the situation. In Britain detailed and specific public intervention has developed over the control of new drug introductions but the choice and determination of industrial research areas remains located within the private sector. This latter characteristic is defended by Maddox in his recent study — 'Pharmaceutical Research and Public Ownership'[7] as being more appropriate for what he terms 'the undeniably speculative character of pharmaceutical research', while Robson has argued that 'a new style of research is needed in the pharmaceutical industry, an obvious prerequisite for which is its removal from the pressures of the private sector'.[8] Before examining the alternative policy options applicable to innovation in the pharmaceutical industry we need to look at the past experience of research and innovation in the UK and the possible influence of public policy on it. The inability to test policies in advance means that we are forced to rely to some extent on history. International comparative studies or the study of trends over time are two common approaches, the difficulty always being to separate the influence of public policy from other factors which may be as, if not more important. However, an analysis of the past pattern of innovation in the industry can at least provide a guide to the degree to which it corresponds or conflicts with health needs. It is this perspective rather than that of export performance and commercial succeess, that is adopted in this study.

The two problems already mentioned — whether too much effort is devoted to wasteful innovation and whether the full spectrum of therapeutic needs is being met — have attracted considerable debate. The reliance on argument by selected examples tends to result in a 'glories' versus 'follies' contest which may be entertaining but is not often very illuminating about the overall pattern of innovation. Let us examine some data which can help to give us some indications of this general picture.

The first question, of course, is what we mean by innovation. I will concentrate on product rather than process innovation and we can define this broadly as being accomplished with the marketing of a product possessing some degree of novelty. This, of course, begs a definition of novelty, and a number of criteria — chemical, pharmaceutical or therapeutic — can be used. Some relative measure of novelty is probably a more useful guide than an absolute definition. Figure 13.2[9] shows the total annual new product introduction in the UK from 1956 to 1974. These include new formulations, combinations and duplications of existing drugs. This overall rate of new product introduction can be compared with the introduction of new single pharmaceutical chemicals (excluding biologicals and new salts of known chemicals) into the UK. These constituted 20 per cent of total product introductions in the UK in 1974. The striking decline in total new product introduction appears to be interrupted only by two flurries of product activity, in the years leading to the start of the Dunlop committee[10] and the implementation of the licensing provisions of the Medicines Act respectively. One can speculate on the extent to which these public interventions inhibited subsequent product introduction or stimulated those immediately beforehand. The decline in overall products is markedly greater than the decline in new single chemicals and without detracting from the importance of innovation in formulation the drop in the number of similar products and combinations probably does not represent any great therapeutic loss. The confusion caused by product proliferation and the doubtful value of many combinations were criticised by a number of authorities during the 1960s.[11]

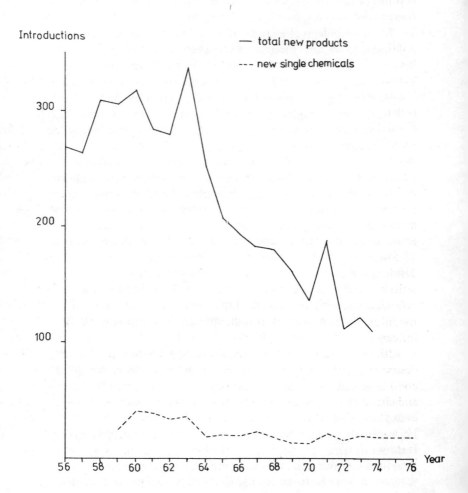

Figure 13.2: Great Britain — Pharmaceutical Products Introduced 1956-76

The decline in new chemicals introduced presents a more serious problem but before considering the significance of this the easy assumption that this decline was solely precipitated by stricter controls on the safety of new drugs must be questioned. In the UK there are signs of a decline from 1960 onwards and similar information for the United States (Figure 13.3) shows a sharp decline from 1960, two years before the Kefauver-Harris Amendments. This has been used by Jennings[12] of the FDA to suggest that an increase in the scientific difficulty of discovering new drugs is a more important factor than regulation in causing this decline. Also worth noting is that regulation of drug safety had been introduced in the 1938 Food, Drug and Cosmetics Act and so the increase in innovation in the 1950s took place within this framework. The decline in new pharmaceutical chemical introduction is a global phenomenon although it has not been smooth or steady. Figure 13.4 shows this and also shows the different pattern among a number of pharmaceutical industries in different countries. The decline in introduction of new pharmaceutical chemicals has been paralleled by an increase in average development time for new products (Figure 13.5) although there is still quite a variation among different products. The lengthening of the R & D process and the decline in introduction reflect a combination of more stringent requirements on safety and efficacy, increasing scientific difficulty in drug discovery and a rise in the costs of research. It is difficult to separate these influences.

Although, in commercial terms, a high rate of innovation may be desirable and a decline is to be deplored, in terms of broader health consideration what is more important is the therapeutic significance and character of innovation rather than simply the rate. An evaluation of the therapeutic gain of new drug introduction in the US was undertaken by the Food and Drug Administration (Figure 13.6). It showed a much greater drop in the less significant innovations than in the modest and important ones. A similar, though less dramatic pattern is shown for the UK (Figure 13.7). These evaluations of therapeutic significance were made for 1959 to 1970 in a survey by clinical experts for the pharmaceutical industry's Office of Health Economics; those for 1971 to 1976 represent the independent evaluations published by Drug and Therapeutics Bulletin, and Medical Letter. Although some relative decline in the innovations offering no or marginal gains can be perceived, these still represent a substantial proportion of introductions. Of particular interest is the large

Figure 13.3: United States — Pharmaceutical Products Introduced 1948-75

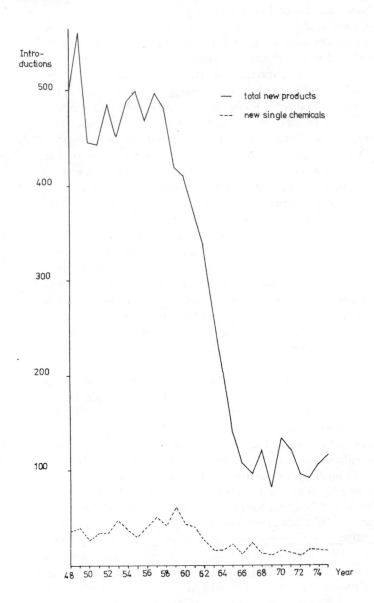

Source: De Haen, New Products Index.

Figure 13.4: Introduction of New Drugs 1961-73 by Nationality of Innovating Firm

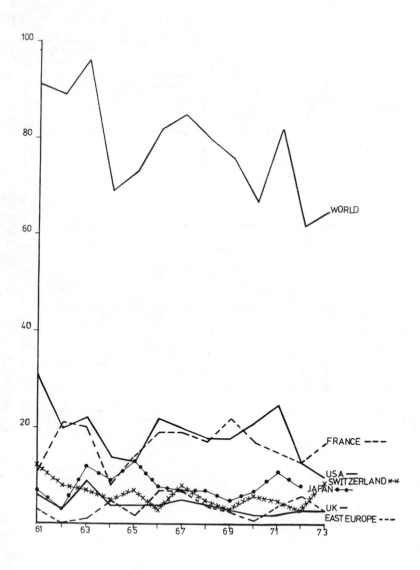

Source: F. Reis-Arndt, *Pharm. Ind.* (1975).

Figure 13.5: Time from First Patent or Publication to UK Marketing

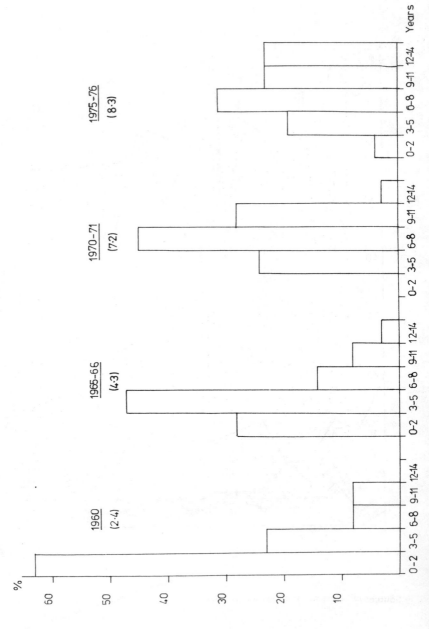

Figure 13.6: United States — Annual Approvals of New Drugs by Degree of Therapeutic Gain 1950-73

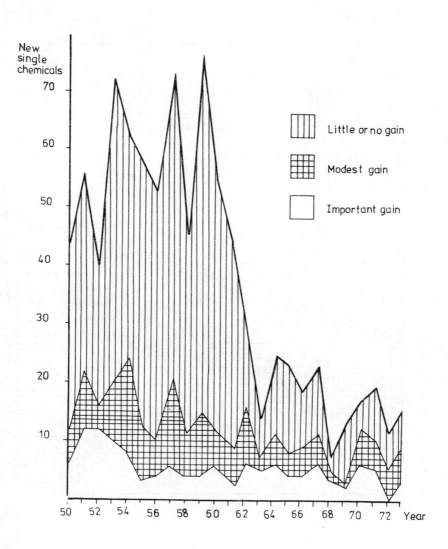

Source: A.M. Schmidt, Statement to Senate Subcommittee on Health (1974).

Figure 13.7: Great Britain — New Drugs Marketed per year
According to Therapeutic Significance 1959-76

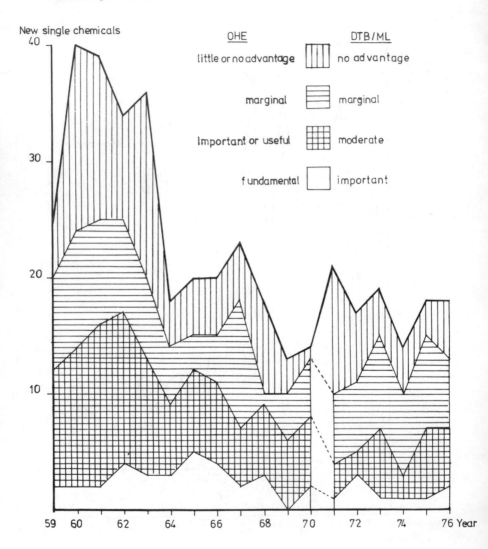

proportion of these in the years 1963 and 1971 which have been referred to as immediately preceding the introduction of certain measures of control. Specific examples of groups of products which have been criticised for their high rate of product introduction include the so called 'Benzodiazepine bonanza'[13] the non-hormonal anti-inflammatories,[14] topical steroids[15] and the many β-blockers.[16] The problem raised by these is not only whether they hinder rather than help effective therapy but whether their development represents a serious misallocation of valuable research resources. Introductions by British owned firms (Figure 13.8) also include a high proportion of products of limited usefulness and it should be pointed out that the evaluations for 1960 to 1970 were acknowledged by those who conducted this study to be biased in favour of British products.[17]

Although there are roughly similar trends to be perceived in the US and the UK, the decline in the US has been sharper. Wardell and Lasagna compared the introduction of new drugs in the two countries and identified the existence of a 'drug lag'. (Figure 13.9) which they considered to stem from the more flexible approach to regulation in the UK. Again the question of the therapeutic significance of this 'lag' arises. Certain important innovations such as disodium cromoglycate were delayed for a considerable time in the US. Conversely Britain's exclusive introductions included a number of products whose benefits were obscure, such as the non-hormonal anti-inflammatory agents as well as products which had to be withdrawn because of unacceptable toxicity, such as ibufenac and practolol.

Interestingly, introductions by the British drug industry show a high rate of withdrawal compared with other countries (Figure 13.10). These withdrawals may be prompted by safety, efficacy or by purely commercial considerations.

As well as changes in the rate and significance of pharmaceutical innovation there are also perceptible shifts in the therapeutic areas covered. Figure 13.11 shows the emergence of cardiovascular drugs (group VII) as a major area. Morbidity and mortality data are provided for comparison but the areas of innovation probably represent a response to a combination of market-pull and technology-push. It is not easy to determine whether there has been a relative shift from innovation in epidemiologically minor areas. Figure 13.12 shows introduction of drugs for diseases of relatively low incidence. There is some decline over the period examined but the main implication is that drugs for genuinely rare disease have remained a consistently

Figure 13.8: New Drugs Discovered by British-owned Firms and Marketed in UK 1960-75 by Therapeutic Significance

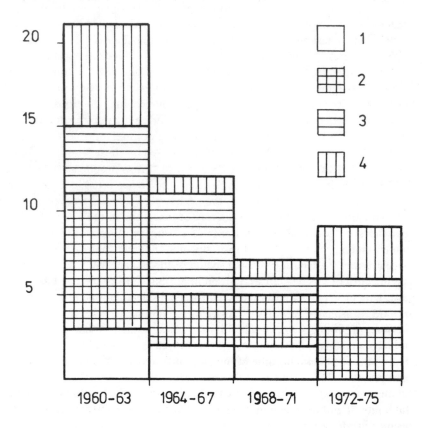

Figure 13.9:First Introduction of New Drugs in Britain and the United States

Country of first marketing	Mutual Introductions		Exclusive Introductions	
	UK	US	UK	UK
1962-71	43	25	77	21
1972-74	12	7	26	10

Source: W.M. Wardell and L. Lasagna, *Regulation and Drug Development*, American Enterprise Institute (1975).

Figure 13.10: Rate of Withdrawal of New Pharmaceutical Chemicals
1961-73

Country of Innovating Firm (Head Office)	% Withdrawal
USA	3.2
France	2.3
W. Germany	7.5
Switzerland	2.5
Italy	1.5
Great Britain	9.6
Scandinavia	5.9

Source: F. Reis-Arndt, *Pharm. Ind.* (1975).

small fraction of innovation. Garattini has referred to the lack of
attention to diseases such as muscular dystrophy, multiple sclerosis
and amyloidosis as examples of the problem.[18] Overall the evidence
on the industry's record of innovation does suggest that while it
has introduced a large number of important therapeutic agents in the
past, these are emerging less frequently. A substantial proportion
of new introductions do not seem to be very useful and uneconomic
disease areas tend to be neglected. Resources devoted to the
industry's research continue to increase (Figure 13.13).

So far this assessment remains one that is internal to pharmaceutical
innovation, but the problem must be placed in the context of
biomedical research in general. Figure 13.14 shows the location of
basic research to be mainly outside the drug industry. In itself this
need not be unacceptable but it is becoming increasingly apparent
that the major diseases that we face, such as cancer and heart disease
are unlikely to be solved by a straightforward chemo-therapeutic fix.
Similar observations have been made regarding rheumatic disease.[19]
This implies a need for a new integration of basic and applied
research and of pharmaceutical with other medical and social sciences.
In policy terms decisions on this would need to be related to the
overall priorities given by government to health research.

...ure 13.11: New Drugs Marketed in Great Britain Classified by Disease Area (ICD 1968 Categories)

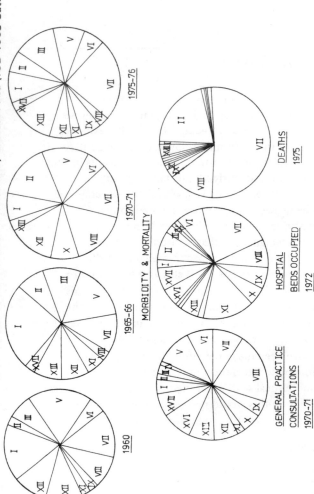

GENERAL PRACTICE
CONSULTATIONS
1970-71

MORBIDITY & MORTALITY

HOSPITAL
BEDS OCCUPIED
1972

DEATHS
1975

WHO International Classification of Disease 1968

Main categories:

I   Infective and Parasitic Diseases (000-136)
II   Neoplasms (140-239)
III Endocrine, Nutritional and Metabolic Diseases (240-279)
IV Diseases of Blood and Blood Forming Organs (280-289)
V   Mental Disorders (290-315)
VI Diseases of the Nervous System and Sense Organs (370-389)
VII Diseases of the Circulatory System (390-458)
VIII Diseases of the Respiratory System (460-519)
IX Diseases of the Digestive System (570-577)
X   Diseases of Genito-Urinary System (580-629)

XI   Complications of Pregnancy, Childbirth and the Puerperium (630-678)
XII Diseases of the Skin and Subcutaneous Tissue (680-709)
XIII Diseases of the Musculo-Skeletal System and Connective Tissue (710-738)
XIV Congenital Anomalies (740-759)
XV Certain Causes of Perinatal Morbidity and Mortality (760-779)
XVI Symptoms and Ill-Defined Conditions (780-796)
XVII Accidents, Poisonings and Violence (800-999)

Figure 13.12: Drugs Introduced for Diseases of Low Incidence in UK (Excluding drugs for cancer and bacterial infection)

1960-2	
D-ALDOSTERONE	Addison's disease
DILOXANIDE	Intestinal amebiasis
ETHOSUXIMIDE	Petit mal
METHIXENE	Parkinsonism
NICLOSAMIDE	Tapeworm
ORPHENADRINE	Parkinsonism
SULFINPYRAZONE	Chronic gout
SULTHIAME	Epilepsy

Total: 8 out of 113 introductions (7.1%)

1971-6	
BENAPRYZINE	Parkinsonism
CARBIDOPA	Parkinsonism
CALCITONIN	Paget's disease of the bone
DESMOPRESSIN	Cranial diabetes insipidus
MEBENDAZOLE	Helmintic infections

Total: 5 out of 107 introductions (4.7%)

(Low incidence = Less than 10 general practice consultations per 1000 population;

Source: Morbidity Statistics from General Practice (1970/71).

Figure 13.13: R & D in UK Pharmaceutical Industry 1967-75

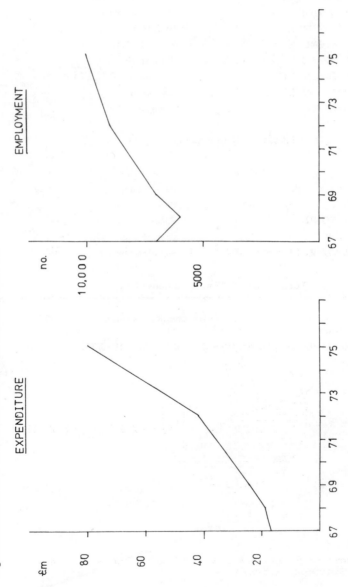

Source: Central Statistical Office, R & D Expenditure and Employment

Figure 13.14a: Expenditure Relating to Medical Research, UK 1973-4

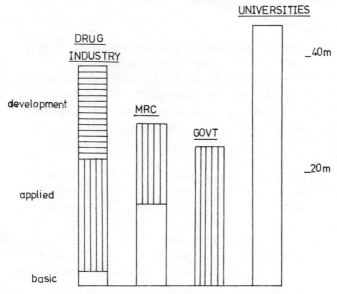

Figure 13.14b: Government R & D Expenditure 1975 (1196.6 m)

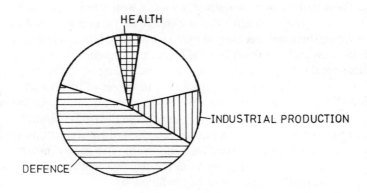

Sources: Central Statistical Office, R & D Expenditure and Employment, 'Statistics of Education'.

Given this background what are the public policy options which have been put forward in recent years? These fall into four main categories.

1. Deregulation

Although it is a popular theme among spokespeople for the industry to criticise the burden of regulations placed upon them by government, in actual fact most accept the need for some regulatory intervention over the safety, efficacy and quality of medicines. The few people who do not, tend to be economists living in the vicinity of Chicago. For example, Sam Peltzman conducted a cost-benefit analysis which concluded that it would cost society less to suffer the occasional thalidomide disaster than to risk a two year delay in a new treatment for TB.[20] He concluded that the United States efficacy requirements introduced in the Kefauver-Harris amendments in 1962 should be abolished. Apart from the basic difficulty of expressing phocomelia in pounds and pence the analysis rests on the assumption that regulation can only inhibit in an unselected manner and that the prescribing of a new drug bears a simple relationship to its quality. The latter owes a good deal more to faith in the 'invisible hand' of the market than to the evidence.

2. Status Quo

Both the Association of the British Pharmaceutical Industry and the present British government agree on the need for some regulatory control over the introduction of new drugs, basically with reference to safety and efficacy. They also agree that the choice of research areas and the direction of innovative activity should remain under the control of a privately owned industry. The recent agreement reached between industry and government rested on just these principles.[21] The dropping of Section 41, the compulsory Licensing provisions, of the Patents Act and the extension of patent cover to 20 years can both function as incentives to innovation in a general sense while the tighter controls over promotion represented a further extension of government power over new product introduction. Naturally within this general policy framework there is considerable room for difference. Some of the issues of contention continue to be the following:

(a) Relative Efficacy Requirements

The ABPI pressed hard for the removal of a relative efficacy requirement in the Medicines Bill when it was passing through Parliament.[22] This would have required the merits of a new drug

relative to those already available to be considered before granting a
licence. The final formulation included in the Act allowed there to be
some consideration of relative efficacy but only in relation to safety.
This clause is somewhat open to interpretation and recently *Drug
and Therapeutics Bulletin* called for an amendment of the law to
strengthen relative efficacy requirements.[23] Naturally it would be
expected that this would not only more strictly control products
coming on to the market but would exert some indirect influence
over research and innovation strategy.

(b) Post – Marketing Surveillance

The adverse effects of practolol have led to suggestions for a more
effective and comprehensive system of monitoring the effects of
new drugs in use.[24]

  The ABPI has been rather hostile to some of these proposals on the
basis that they would discourage doctors from prescribing new drugs
and hence act as an obstacle to innovation.[25]

(c) Classification of Medicines

The McGregor committee functioned for a number of years as a
body which classified new medicines according to their therapeutic
value. The industry was not in favour of such a procedure and the
McGregor committee was finally dissolved.[26] This amounted to the
removal of an influence on the market for new drugs.

  Nevertheless, in spite of these major issues of contention
concerning the control of innovation, none of them challenges the
basic philosophy of direct controls only over the innovative output
of the industry while leaving direct determination of research policy
to the industry itself.

3. Limited State Ownership and Control

General incentives to innovate do not necessarily lead in socially
desirable directions – as the Public Accounts Committee observed in
1960. The first voluntary Price Regulation Scheme differentiated in
favour of new drugs by not subjecting them to price control for a
few years after introduction but it was later felt that this simply
encouraged unnecessary product introductions.[27]

  This poses the question as to whether the government should
not exert a more direct influence on the determination of research
policy in the industry. The Labour Party's working group on the
drug industry suggested that one major firm should be taken into

public ownership and that Planning Agreements should be adopted with the industry as a whole. This would imply that the Government could then exert a controlling influence over the research policy of one firm and some influence (along with trade-unions) over the general volume and direction of R & D in the industry as a whole. The proposals probably embody two distinct approaches – one simply seeing a need to fill the gap left by private industry and to conduct research into 'unprofitable' areas; the other seeing this limited intervention as part of a strategic process of bringing the industry fully under public control.[28]

4. Full State-Ownership and Control

The proposals for full state ownership, made for example by the Haslemere Group[29] and John Robson[30] rest on the view that such a basis would be required for a rational integration of the industry's research with the nation's overall health research. This position argues that the private direction of research and innovation is not in the general social interest and direct public control of both the inputs to and outputs of technological change in the drug industry is required. Although arguing for integration, it is emphasised that this does not necessarily correspond to a simple centralisation of research policy making.

These various policy options represent different approaches to the fundamental problem with which I opened; that of controlling technological change in the social interest. Given the recent pattern of pharmaceutical innovation, it would seem that policy change rather than preservation of the status quo is required. Of particular importance in this regard is the separation of public control over innovative output from the private promotion and choice of research. The policies which seek to bridge this gap are those that merit more serious attention than they are often given.

Notes

*This area of investigation was suggested to me by Professor D.G. Wibberley, Head of the Department of Pharmacy, University of Aston, whose continuous encouragement and advice has been invaluable

1. *Industrial Innovation – Strategies and Risks* (Science Policy Foundation, Hilton Hotel, January 1977).
2. H. Tandy, *Financial Times*, 20 June 1977, Supplement on the Chemical Industry.
3. M.S. Baram, Technology Assessment and Social Control', *Science*, 180

(1973), p.465.
4. J. Spink, *Pharmaceutical Journal*, 13 September 1975, p.243.
5. Labour Party: *Discussion document on the Pharmaceutical Industry* (1976).
6. NEDO, *Focus on Pharmaceuticals* (HMSO, 1972).
7. J. Maddox, *Pharmaceutical Research and Public Ownership* (ABPI, 1975).
8. J. Robson, *'Take a Pill' – the Drug Industry – Private or Public* (Communist Party pamphlet, 1972).
9. Overall product introductions from DHSS; New single chemicals from NEDO; Pharmaceutical Index; Pharmaceutical Journal.
10. The Dunlop Committee (Committee on the Safety of Drugs) commenced work in January 1964. The licensing provisions of the Medicines Act came into force in September 1971 (licenses of right were granted to all products marketed at least one month previously).
11. By, for example, the McGregor Committee on the Classification of Proprietary Preparations.
12. J. Jennings, 'Government Regulations and Drug Development: FDA' in *Drug Discovery* (1972), p.247.
13. P. Tyrer, *The Lancet*, (21 September 1974), p.709.
14. *British Medical Journal*, (10 January 1976), p.59.
15. *Drug and Therapeutics Bulletin*, 15, p.59.
16. *Drug and Therapeutics Bulletin*, 14 (17), (1976), p.65.
17. NEDO, *Innovative Activity in the Pharmaceutical Industry* (HMSO, 1973).
18. S. Garattini, *Impact of Science on Society*, XXV (3) (1975).
19. *British Medical Journal* (10 January 1976).
20. S. Peltzman, *Regulation of Pharmaceutical Innovation* (American Enterprise Institute, 1974).
21. *Pharmaceutical Journal*, 7 (May 1977).
22. R. Lang, *The Politics of Drugs* (Saxon House, 1972).
23. *Drug and Therapeutics Bulletin*, 14 (17) (1976), p.65.
24. C.T. Dollery and M.D. Rawlings, British Medical Journal, 1 (1977), p.96.
25. A.B. Wilson, 'New Medicines', paper given at Industrial Innovation – Strategies and Risks, Conference, 1977.
26. *Guardian*, 14 May 1974.
27. R. Lang, *op.cit.*
28. S. Holland, *The Socialist Challenge* (Quartet, 1975).
29. Haslemere Group, *Who Needs the Drug Companies* (Third World Publications, 1976).
30. J. Robson, *op. cit.*

14 NEW DRUGS FOR PATIENTS

Brian W. Cromie

Introduction

The pharmaceutical industry exists to invent, manufacture and provide new therapeutic agents, ensuring that doctors have information about them and that the medicines are available for patients who need them.

The pharmaceutical industry in the UK fulfils these objectives and, additionally, makes an enormous contribution to the economy of the country, despite increasingly restrictive controls and an environment of misinformed, emotive criticism.

Research

In order to invent medicines with therapeutic advantages, the industry conducts research. Research starts as an idea, takes shape in synthetic chemistry laboratories, goes through toxicity testing, pharmacology, volunteer studies in man and extensive clinical trials. At every stage in the process there are hurdles and at every stage decisions have to be taken.

(a) UK Success

The pharmaceutical industry is world-wide and has produced virtually all the effective medicines used by doctors today. However, pharmaceutical research in the UK has been particularly successful with semi-synthetic penicillins, beta-blockers, sodium cromoglycate, potent topical steroids, salbutamol and, more recently, cimetidine for peptic ulceration and labetalol for hypertension. All made significant contributions to improved patient care and all came from UK pharmaceutical research.

(b) Reasons for Success

Why is a competitive, private-enterprise pharmaceutical industry successful, particularly in the UK?

The main reason is basically team-work of competent scientists working together towards a common goal, who are not side-tracked by individual interests and hobby horses and who are led by research directors who are prepared to make decisions. Few people outside research realize the enormity of these decisions, which involve

undertaking multi-million pound ventures or, more difficult,
abandoning projects that have been followed for years and taken up
hundreds of scientist man-years. In his attempt to save our heritage
of beautiful houses in an era of CTT, Lord Tavistock[1] recently said that
'a house cannot be run by a civil servant'. In a similar way, civil servants
could never accept the responsibility of decisions which have to be
taken for research to be successful and cost-effective. Perhaps that
is why state-sponsored industries produce loss-making successes like
'Concorde', while our pharmaceutical industry produces profitable
products that also benefit patients and help the country's ailing
economy.

There is no doubt that individual responsibility in a competitive
industry sharpens the mind wonderfully but there are other reasons for
the success of the pharmaceutical industry in the UK and many of
these lie in the NHS. Firstly, we have a reputation for high calibre
clinical work, secondly there is a wide-spread recognition in our
hospitals of a responsibility to foster clinical research and thirdly we
pay our doctors so poorly in comparison with American and European
colleagues that the industry can afford to employ amongst the best of
our doctors. Companies in this country are thus able to get the best
clinical advice and support in the world.

(c) UK Problems

The successes of pharmaceutical research in the UK has not, however,
been obtained without problems. A major problem is cost. As
therapeutic advances become more difficult and as regulations
increase, it becomes more difficult and more time-consuming and
expensive to develop the products now required by today's clinicians.
The average figures suggest a ten-year project involving nearly 10,000
compounds and costing £10m to £15m to develop a new compound.
All that has to be paid for, which a recent review[2] quotes as high risk
capital with an average 3 to 4 per cent return and a pay-back 20
years.

This investment can only come from sales of today's drugs but the
prices of these are rigidly controlled. In the past ten years, the
profitability of the pharmaceutical industry has fallen to 15 per cent or
lower,[2] while the average for UK industry generally has increased from
13 to 17 per cent. The cost of today's drugs in relation to their cost of
manufacture or of the research which produced them is all quite
immaterial; if therapeutic advances are to continue, then today's
sales must pay for tomorrow's improved therapy and the research

which produces it.

It would, of course be reasonable if all of the increased research costs were productive but a recent review of regulations emanating from the FDA[3] — that fount of pharmaceutical regulations — suggests that many produced loss rather than gain. Certainly, the latest crop dealing with GLP (Good Laboratory Practice) is merely an increase in documentation which will cause an estimated increase in costs of 25 to 30 per cent. This represents a corresponding decrease in innovative research with no balancing gain.

Regulations are world-wide but a problem which is more particular to the UK is having to work in an environment of uninformed anti-vivisection activities. Nobody wants to use animals in research where there are alternatives, as these would be standardised, reproducible and cheaper. If this was recognised by freak groups, they could use their time constructively in trying to prevent Governments asking for unnecessary animal tests instead of trying to burn down laboratories, such as mine at Milton Keynes, which was particularly designed to encourage early human metabolic studies and prevent studies in irrelevant species and yet was the object of two arson attempts by groups who even appeared to get covert support from authorities when caught. It is problems like these and the peripheral ones, such as pay policies that prevent rewarding individual merit, which make the UK successes in pharmaceutical research all the more remarkable and we must accordingly be grateful.

Distribution

As was stated by way of introduction, the pharmaceutical industry exists to invent, manufacture and provide new therapeautic agents. Let us consider the provision, on demand, of medicines of guaranteed quality in the manner laid down by Government licences, at reasonable prices.

(a) Availability

Whatever other problems may have arisen from time to time in the NHS with strikes, pickets, 'emergency-only' policies or what-have-you, the medicines produced by the UK pharmaceutical industry have always been available.

Irrespective of external industrial disputes, the pharmaceutical industry has shown a flexibility of switching staff and distribution methods to ensure that medicines always got through. In a similar way, factory fires or the three strikes within the industry (van drivers in one company, electricians in another and chemical workers in a third) over the last 25 years have always been overcome by co-operation between companies and demands for medicines have been met.

(b) Controlled Quality

The medicines supplied have also been of guaranteed quality. They are manufactured under conditions of GMP (Good Manufacturing Practice), supervised by DHSS inspectorate. The manufacturer's trade mark is the surety that all products released for sale under that mark will have equivalent clinical performance under similar conditions. A reassurance which cannot, of course, be extended to other formulations of the same active ingredients. The medicines also come from the manufacturer in tested packages with patient warnings, where necessary, and with a batch number to allow recall should any error in manufacture or packing occur.

It is unfortunate that, in this country, we have not followed the more general European and American practice of giving patients their medicines in 'mint condition' and with all the necessary warnings, etc. on the package itself. We allow our pharmacists to remove tablets and capsules from a tested and licensed container to a different container without any supervision of the methods of transfer. This also divorces the medicament from any patient warning and no separate leaflet will ever be as effective as wording on the container itself. It also removes the batch number, so that no recall system can go beyond the retail pharmacist. It is surely time that the UK abandoned this medieval system of dispensing and ensured that patients received their medicines in the 'original pack' from the manufacturer, with all the safety and control elements which that entails.

(c) Reasonable Prices

Medicines are also available in the UK at reasonable prices or rather at prices which the DHSS considers reasonable. There is no question that the price of a medicine should merely relate to its ingredient and manufacturing cost any more than a Rembrandt is valued at the cost of canvas and paint or advanced computers at the cost of combined parts.

The cost must bear the total investment of a continuing, research-based industry, which is making a major contribution to health and to the economy of the country. The DHSS, therefore, bear these points in mind when each company produces a full Annual Financial Return and forecast for the Government to scrutinise and

to consider in an ongoing review of prices and profits under the
recently re-named Pharmaceutical Price Regulation Scheme (PPRS).

Despite this recognition that the UK must make some
contribution to world-wide R & D from which it benefits, this
country basically operates a 'cheap-drugs policy', being amongst the
cheapest in Europe and resulting in a fall in the total NHS bill from
11.2 per cent to 8.4 per cent for medicines in the last ten years,
while the volume of prescriptions has increased by 50 per cent. A
true example of increased productivity of lower relative costs!

We live in cost-conscious times and must try and get the most for
every taxed pound that goes into the health services. This means
bolstering primary care with effective medicines at an average of
200p per prescription, as compared to a hospital stay costing about
£200 for an equivalent time.

Information to Doctors

The third part of the introductory triad, after invention and making
available, was ensuring that doctors have information about
medicines. Information must be accurate but it must also be
understandable and disseminated by an effective system, as no single
patient will benefit from a therapeutic advance, however
significant, unless his doctor is aware of that advance and knows how
to use it.

(a) Effective

Whatever other comments people may make about the information
dissemination system of the UK pharmaceutical industry, nobody
can deny that it is effective. Every survey has shown that the
industry is the most important aspect in knowing that drugs are
available, while other influences are more important for actual
usage.[4]

Our own investigations suggest that the average family doctor
will know about an advance in surgery that might be of help to his
patients after seven or eight years but 80 per cent will know of an
advance in medical therapeautics within nine months; what is
more, they will understand it.

To some extent, every public gets the advertisements it deserves
and doctors are no exception. Extensive pre-testing is carried out
to ensure that the basic message about a new medicine is understood
and remembered. This aspect should always be considered before
anybody comments on a particular advertisement; apart from

excesses of bad taste, the first question should be 'Has it done its job?'

(c) Controlled

The pharmaceutical manufacturer must be the final source of knowledge of his formulated medicines but he still has to work within very tight limits to achieve the effectiveness just referred to.

The basic facts in all advertisements must comply with a data sheet which will now be part of the Government-approved product licence. The contents must also comply with a Code of Practice, drawn up by the industry in conjunction with the DHSS and the BMA and any breaches of the Code will be judged by a committee under an independent QC with a membership including an independent GP and consultant. Similarly, representatives must comply with the Code and will now have to limit their calls to three times per year and to show an official data sheet before discussing any pharmaceutical product.

Finally, the total amount of money spent on information dissemination and related services, drawn together under the blanket term 'promotion', is subject to strict Governmental control by means of the PPRS and the independently-audited Annual Financial Return submitted by each company each year to the DHSS.

(c) Multi-Purpose

Although the emphasis on the information-related services is generally on the data given to doctors, they are really much broader than that. In the first place, discussion between practising doctors and industry representatives gives a dialogue with practical information coming back to the manufacturers. Many modifications in dosage, packaging, presentation or formulation have originated from such a dialogue.

In the second place, the company hears about adverse reactions and follows-up and reports all that come to their knowledge, so that more adverse reaction reports eventually get to the CSM through action of the pharmaceutical industry than by any other method.

After the practolol episode, it is clear that no amount of pre-clinical testing can prevent the possibility of patient hazard and that our greatest guarantee of limiting toxic effects is good adverse-reaction reporting. To put the matter into perspective, the latest review suggests that non-intravenous drugs probably contributed significantly to mortality in 1 in 50,000 hospitalised patients,[5] so the risks for the average patient are minute. Nevertheless, no effective drug is absolutely safe and both doctors and the pharmaceutical

industry are at fault if they suggest otherwise. There must always be a
recognized balance of benefit to risk, which should also be accepted
by patients. For some odd reason, patients appear to accept a risk to
benefit chance with surgery but expect medicines to be completely
safe — further education is clearly needed.

Whatever the patient attitude, it is certain that the pharmaceutical
industry and the medical profession must work together to improve
the reporting of adverse reactions, particularly with new drugs, and to
obtain total recall in the unlikely event of problems arising.

In my view this will not be achieved in a realistic way with
'monitored release' or special prescription pads, as have been
suggested. The greatest hope lies in the normal prescribing of new
medicines in original packs with a detachable label, which the pharmacist
can then stick onto the FP 10. This would allow a data base, with
only minor modifications to the present Prescription Pricing Authority
(PPA),[6] so that hypotheses on toxicity could be tested and, if
necessary, doctors and patients warned and the drug effectively
and rapidly withdrawn.

All of this lies in the future but it does illustrate the wider role,
which can be played under the general heading of providing information
to doctors about drugs available for their use.

Conclusions

The health services in the UK are becoming increasingly expensive
and have increased by 30 per cent as a proportion of the country's
GNP in the last ten years and overmanning is such that the Secretary
of State for Social Services has stated that, if the trend of the past
twenty years continues, every member of the population would be
an employee of the Health Service by the year 2100.[7] Despite this,
the morale of the doctors and nurses in the hospitals is low and the
standards of primary medical care are falling.

Against this background of other aspects of health care, the
pharmaceutical industry in the UK stands out as a shining example
of successful innovation and higher productivity at lower costs. It
is not a philanthropic organisation but neither is it an industry of
uncontrolled profits. In fact, it is the most controlled industry in the UK
and it can only continue successfully if, within those controls, it
invents and produces medicines with therapeutic advantages that
doctors are informed about and find useful for their patients. It is a
system that has worked in the past to the enormous benefit of
patients and also to the economy of the country. If it is to continue,

its value must be recognised and cherished.

One measure of recognition by the Government is the recent Patent Bill, which disallowed compulsory licences, but such recognition is not general in the public domain and some people still wish to make dramatic changes. They would do so, not just at their own peril, but at the risk of the population and the economy of the UK.

Notes

1. *The Times*, 13 June 1977.
2. 'Pharmaceutical Industry Dynamics and Outlook to 1985' (Health Industries Resource Dept., Stanford Reference Institute, 1977), and 'Intangible Capital and Rates of Return' (Clarkson, American Enterprise Instituting, 1977).
3. G.F. Roll, 'Of Politics and Drug Regulations', (The Center for the Study of Drug Development, University of Rochester Medical Center, PS − 7701, January 1977).
4. 'Prescribing in General Practice', 1976 Roy. Coll, Gen. Practit.
5. 'Deaths Due to Drug Treatment', Editorial, *British Medical Journal*, 1 (1977), p. p.1492.
6. R.I. Tricker, *Report of the Inquiry into the Prescription Pricing Authority* (Oxford Centre for Management Studies, 1977).
7. *Fortune*, April 1977, p.139.

CONTRIBUTORS

Sir Douglas Black is Emeritus Professor of Medicine in the University of
Manchester and President of the Royal College of Physicians.

Dr'G.P. Thomas is Fellow of Linacre College, Oxford and Deputy Director,
Department for External Studies, University of Oxford.

Alan Williams is Professor at the Department of Economics, University
of York.

The Radical Statistics Health Group is an informal group of medical
statisticians and doctors concerned with the political use of medical
statistics and health information.

A.T. Altschul is Professor of Nursing Studies at the University of
Edinburgh.

Dr Patricia E. O'Connell, SRN, is Lecturer in Charge, Health Visitor
Courses at the University of Southampton.

Pat Gordon was Secretary of City and Hackney Community Health
Council from 1974 to March 1978.

Ernest Braun is Director of the Technology Policy Unit, The University
of Aston in Birmingham.

D. Collingridge is Lecturer at the Technology Policy Unit, University of
Aston in Birmingham; *Mr K. Edwards* and *Mr J. McEvoy* are research
students in the Unit.

Dr L.S. Levy is Head of the Industrial Toxicology Unit, the Department
of Safety and Hygiene, the University of Aston in Birmingham,

O.L. Wade, MD, FRCP, is Professor of Therapeutics and Clinical
Pharmacology, at the University of Birmingham Medical School.

Peter A. Parish, MD FRCGP is Professor at the Division of Clinical
Pharmacy, the Welsh School of Pharmacy, UWIST, Cardiff.

H.F. Steward is Research Fellow in the Department of Pharmacy of the
Technology Policy Unit, the University of Aston in Birmingham.

Dr Brian W. Cromie, FRCP, is Chairman of Hoechst Pharmaceuticals,
Hounslow, Middlesex.

INDEX

Aberdare Health Centre 59
abortion 64-5
Acts: Food, Drugs, and Cosmetics
Act 137; Health and Safety at
Work Act, 1974 111; Health
Visiting and Social Work (Training)
Act 50; LAS Services Act 50;
Medicines Act 132, 135; National
Insurance Act, 1911 16
American National Institute of
Occupational Safety and Health
(NIOSH) 103, 104
Ames mutation system 111
Association of the British Pharmaceut-
ical Industry 119, 120, 150-1

Barem, M.S. 132-3
Bills: James White Abortion Amendment Bill 64; Medical Practitioners
(Restriction of Right to Prescribe)
Bill, 1976 122; NHS Reorganisation
Bill 60; Patent Bill 162
blood lead levels 77-89; and daily
assimilation of lead 91; in adult
urban males 82; in adults 79-80,
82; in children 78-9; in poor
Mexicans 81; 'natural' 81; see also
lead
Briggs, Professor Asa 39
Briggs Committee on Nursing 39, 42,
43, 44, 54
British Medical Association (BMA)
119, 160
British National Formulary (BNF)
118, 122, 124

cadmium 72-3, 74
Canada see North America
cancer 100-14; causes of 101;
characteristics of 100-1; factors
in the development of 102-3;
incidence of 101-2; see also
carcinogens
Caplan, G. 53
carcinogens: animal studies of 109-11,
112; epidemiological studies of
108-9, 112; industrial 103-13;
short-term tests of 111;

Threshold Limit Values (TLV) of
105, 107
carcinogens: arsenic 106; asbestos 103,
106; bis (chloromethyl) ether 107;
nickel 107; radiations 106, 107;
soot 106; vinyl chloride monomer
107
Cartwright, A. 123
Chief Scientist's Research Committee
(CSRC) 21
City and East London Area Health
Authority 62
Cochrane, Professor A.L. 24n4
Community Health Councils (CHC)
59-68; and abortion services 64-5;
and complaints 65-7; and hospital
closures 60-1; and information to
Health Authorities 63-5; and
information to public 61-3; and
nutrition 62-3; and services to
elderly 63-4; beginnings of 60;
responsibilities of 60-1
Community Health Councils (CHC):
City and Hackney 61, 62, 64-5;
Halton 66-7; Haringey 61; Leeds
67; Liverpool Central and
Southern 66; St Thomas's 62;
South Tyneside 67; Tower
Hamlets 67; Wandsworth and East
Merton 58, 59, 63, 64; Worthing
63-4
Comroe, J.H. 14
Cook, J.W. 107
Council for the Education and Training
of Health Visitors (CETHV) 50-2,
54, 55
Court Committee on Child Health
Services 54

DDT, distribution of in human body
fat 83
Department of Education and Science,
Science Vote 15, 16
Department of Health and Social
Security (DHSS) 118, 127-8, 130,
158-9, 160; and Chief Scientist
20-1; and research 15-24
Department of the Environment 92